Health Policy and Strategies

By

Rajendra Pratap Gupta

PREFACE

Health is crucial for every individual, family, organization, and nation. We cannot have a prosperous and happy nation without healthy individuals. Delivery of healthcare depends upon governance and financing to start with, which, in turn, depends on the country's policies. Finally, everything boils down to the health policy! If the policies are not aligned with the needs of the people, people will never be healthy or prosperous. This puts the spotlight on health policymaking, i.e., the health policy process.

For India, it is more important to have the right health policies in place given the mix of the population; India is referred to as a young country with an average age being 29 years, but we also have over 120 million senior citizens. In the next twenty-five years, one out of five Indians will be senior citizens. So, it is important to study.

What is the process for making the health policy?

What are the components of Health policy?

What are the problems in each of the identified components of Health policy?

What are the key actors involved in the policy-making process for the national health policy 2017?

How can we improve the health policymaking process in India?

This research has been done to study and make recommendations for improving the policymaking process, which will lead to the formulation of long-term, inclusive, and robust health policies resulting in increasing longevity and a healthy working population.

The study gives a historical backdrop of policies regarding health and the organizational structure and studies the key influencers in policymaking. The study makes recommendations based on inputs from every level in healthcare delivery – urban-rural, public-private, clinicians – and non-clinicians. I am sure these recommendations will help the country define a policymaking process and help policymakers make their policy process inclusive and robust, eventually resulting in better health outcomes.

For me, this doctorate is an important milestone. I continued my advocacy efforts for India to draft its national health policy considering the developments post the 2002 National Health Policy. The magic moment came in 2013 when I was tasked to draft the vision and policies for the current government. While I had the good fortune of drafting policies across sectors, my work in the National Health Policy and National Education Policy was the most fulfilling. When I reflect on those policies, I can safely say that drafting policies is much easier than doing a doctorate in the policymaking process. More so, since such a study- research has not been undertaken on the health policy process in India. Also, this research was a massive effort, and I had to accommodate other important assignments along with completing this research.

However, this research study became easier due to a great professional environment at the IIHMR University with some of the most exemplary academics who kept the momentum.

I must mention **Mr. Ashok Agarwal** for igniting the spark to do this research, **Dr. P.R. Sodani** for his valued guidance and support, and the friendly **Dr. S.D. Gupta**, **Dr. D.K. Mangal**, **Dr. Arindam Das**, **Dr. J.P Singh**, and others who stood by me to complete this. I am sure it will help improve the policymaking in the times ahead.

Place: Jaipur

Date: (Rajendra   Pratap

LIST OF ABBREVIATIONS

A
AAAQ- Availability, Accessibility, Acceptability, and Quality
AHPI- Association of Healthcare Providers
AIDS – Acquired Immune Deficiency Syndrome
AIIMS- All India Institute of Medical Sciences
ANM - Auxiliary Nurse Midwife
ASHA – Accredited Social Health Activist
ASSOCHAM- Associated Chambers of Commerce and Industry of India
AYUSH - Ayurveda, Yoga and Naturopathy, Unani, Siddha, and Homeopathy
B
BCG- Bacille Calmette-Guerin
BRIC – Brazil Russia, India China
C
CAG – Comptroller and Auditor General
CDP- Community Development Program
CHW - Community Health Workers
CSSM- Child Survival and Safe Motherhood
CBHI- Central Bureau of Health Intelligence
CII- Confederation of Indian Industry
CSOs – Civil Society Organizations
D
DALYs- Disability-Adjusted Life Years
DAVP – Directorate of Advertising and Visual Publicity
DGHS - Directorate General of Health Services
DDT- Dichlorodiphenyltrichloroethane
DHKI- District Health Knowledge Institutes
DDAP- Drug De-addiction Programme, Revised in 1993
E
EAG- Empowered Action Group
F

FRCH- Foundation for Research in Community Health
FICCI- Federation of Indian Chambers of Commerce and Industry
FP- Family Planning
FPAI- Family Planning Association of India
FYP - Five Year Plan

G

GNI- Gross National Income
GDP- Gross Domestic Product
GII- Gender-Inequality Index
GDI- Gender Development Index
GoI- Government of India

H

HRH- Human resources in Health
HLEG- High-Level Expert Group
HWC's - Health and Wellness Centres
HIV – Human Immunodeficiency Virus
HDI- Human Development Index
HDRO- Human Development Report Office

I

IAS- Indian Administrative Service
IPS- Indian Police Service
ICDS- Integrated Child Development Services
IDSP- Integrated Disease Surveillance Projects
ICPD - International Conference on Population and Development
IUCD - Intra-Uterine Contraceptive Device
ICSSR – Indian Council of Social Science Research
ICMR- Indian Council of Medical Research
IMR – Infant Mortality Rate

M

MDGs – Millennium Development Goals
MNP – Minimum Needs Programme
MPW- Multi-Purpose Workers
MoHFW- Ministry of Health and Family Welfare
MDM- Mid-Day Meal

M&E – Monitoring and Evaluation

N

NFHS- National Family Health Survey

NACO- National AIDS Control Organization

NHA- National Health Authority

NIHFW- National Institute of Health and Family Welfare

NHSRC - National Health Systems Resource Centre

NMSC – National Medical Service Corporation

NRHM- National Rural Health Mission

NIH- National Institute of Health

NMEP- National Malaria Eradication Program

NHP- National Health Policy

NCHRH- National Council for Human Resources in Health

NHRDA- National Health Regulatory and Development Authority

NDRDA- National Drug Regulatory and Development Authority

NHPPT- National Health Promotion and Protection Trust

NFCP -National Filaria Control Programme

NGEP- National Guinea Worm Eradication Programme

NLEP -National Leprosy Eradication Programme

NVBDCP- National Vector Borne Disease Control Programme

NGCP- National Goitre Control Programme

NCCP- National Cancer Control Programme /NPPCC- National Programme for Prevention and Control of Cancer

NPCB- National Programme for Control of Blindness

NCRP- National Cancer Registry Programme

NMHP - National Mental Health Programme

NGCP- National Goitre Control Programme was renamed NIDDCP- National Iodine Deficiency Disorder Control Programme

NACP- National AIDS Control Programme

NPCTOD -National Programme for Control and Treatment of Occupational Diseases

NPPCD - National Programme for Prevention and Control of Deafness

NTCP - National Tobacco Control Programme

NPPCF - National Programme for Prevention and Control of Fluorosis

NPHCE - National Programme for Health Care in Elderly

NRR – Net Replacement Rate
NITI- National Institution for Transforming India
NCH- National Commission for Homoeopathy
NHM- National Health Mission
NHUM- National Urban Health Mission
NCD- Non-Communicable Diseases
NGO- Non-Government Organization
NHWA- National Health Workforce Account
NTC -National TB Control Programme

O

OOP- Out-of-Pocket
OOPE- Out-of-Pocket Expenditure

P

PGDA- Program on the Global Demography of Aging
PMP- Policy-Making Process
PMSSY- Pradhan Mantri Swasthya Suraksha Yojana
PHU- Primary Health Unit
PHC – Primary Health Care
PM-JAY- Pradhan Mantri Jan Arogya Yojana
PPP- Private -Public Partnership

R

RNTCP- Revised National TB Control Programme
RCH- Reproductive and Child Health Programme
RGNDWM- Rajiv Gandhi National Drinking Water Mission
RMNCH+A- Reproductive, Maternal, Newborn, Child Health and Adolescent

S

SARS- Severe Acute Respiratory Syndrome
SDG- Sustainable Development Goals
SA- South Africa

T

TB- Tuberculosis
TRIPS – Trade-related Aspects of Intellectual Property Rights

U

UNICEF- United Nations International Children's Emergency Fund

UHC – Universal Health Coverage

USA- United States of America

UIP- Universal Immunization Programme

UPHC- Urban Primary Health Centres

UN- United Nations

V

VBDP- Voluntary Blood Donation Programme

W

WHO – World Health Organization

Contents

Introduction 1
    Research Background – Rationale 3
    Scope of the Study 3
    Purpose of the Study 3
    Research Questions 4
    Structure of the Study 4
    Policymaking 4
    Policy Arena 7
    Decisions on Policy Changes 7
    Challenges 8

Literature Review 10
    Prioritizing Health 10
    Health - Economic Growth and Development 10
    Health Indicators - National Family Health Survey (NFHS) 12
        The National Family Health Survey 2015-2016 12
        National Family Health Survey – 2019-21 13
    Evolution of Health Planning and Policies 15
    Constitution of India & Health 16
    Healthcare Policies 20
    Administrative Set-up, Financing and Management of Healthcare in India 22
        NITI Aayog 22
        Administrative set-up 22
        Ayushman Bharat Scheme 26
        Health and Wellness Centres (HWCs) 28
        Healthcare Financing 28
    Universal Health Coverage (UHC) 29
    Foundation of the National Medical Service Corporation (NMSC) 30
    Further emphasis on evidence-based health policy and research on healthcare 30
    Human Resource for Health 31
    Health Policy and Plans 32
    National Health Policy 2002 44
    HLEG Report 2010 52
    Various Committees on Health 55

Health and Human Development Report 2020 57
National Health Policy 2017 58
Focus areas of NHP-2017 60
National Rural Health Mission 65
National Urban Health Mission (NUHM) 67
National Health Mission (NHM) 68
Sustainable Development Goals – SDGs 70
Economic Survey – 2020-21 70
Challenges in Health Policy Making Process in India 72
Relevance of evidence-based policy making to the Indian context 73
Challenges 73

Methodology 77
Research Design 77
Study Population 77
Exclusion and Inclusion Criteria 78
Geographies Covered 78
Sampling Method 79
Study Sample Size 80
Duration of the Study 80
Data Collection 80
Questions asked in the Survey 81
Statistical Analysis 84
Findings 84
Quantitative Results 85
Qualitative Results 158

Discussion 176
Strengths 184
Recommendations 185
State Health Policy 187
Awareness 187
Communication and Technology 187
Inclusive Approach 187
Quality of Data 188
Evidence-Based Policymaking – Research 188
Capacity Building 188
Impact Assessment – M&E 188

Formalizing the Policymaking Process 189
Bibliography 190

Introduction

Generally, the health policies are considered formal, written documents, rules, and guidelines that reflect the decision of policymakers about the steps needed to strengthen the health system and lead to improved health (Gilson, 2012, p. 28). A policy is not just an intervention; it is the primary impetus for the intervention and how changes are initiated (Chhetri and Zacarias, 2021). If we review the ten major public health achievements of the twentieth century, policy change was the reason behind each of them, be it the laws regarding the use of seat belt or regulations governing permissible workplace exposures (Brownson, Chriqui, & Stamatakis, 2009).

Health policies address health concerns and determine what, when, where, and how an individual obtains health care services. They are designed to safeguard and improve community health, and this frequently entails advocating for and bringing about policy measures (De Leeuw et al., 2014). To enhance community health, practitioners, innovators, and public health thinkers must commit to policy reforms that create and promote a health-enhancing environment (Johnson SA, 2009). Health policy is the starting point to bring about a change in the situation (Srinivasan, 1995).

India did not have a National Health Policy for thirty-five years post-independence; till then, the policy directions related to health were drawn from the plan documents developed by the planning commission of India. Post the 80's India has drafted national health policies almost every two decades; The National Health Policy of 1983 and the National Health Policy of 2002, and these two policies have steered the health sector's approach through the Five-Year Plans. If we consider the time lag between the three health policies, the first national health policy came thirty-five years after independence, second national health policy came after eighteen years and the third national health policy came after fourteen years. So, there was no consistency in the timeline for review or formulation of the national health policy. The national scenario with regards to health has changed in four significant ways fourteen years since the second health policy:

- *To start with, health priorities have become diverse, and its spectrum has widened. Although maternal and infant mortality has decreased significantly, the burden of non-communicable illnesses increased along with a few infectious diseases.*

- *The second massive change is the health care sector's growth, which is expected to grow in double digits.*
- *The third development is the increasing percentage of catastrophic spending (out of pocket) because of the health care expenses, which is believed to be amongst the primary cause for poverty.*
- *Fourth, substantial financial support from the government has enabled higher budgetary spending on health. Hence, a new health policy that addresses these dynamic changes is needed* (Ministry of Health & Family Welfare, Government of India, 2017).

India had made a significant commitment to increasing investments towards health care in the last five-year plan i.e., 12th FYP. It made a strong case for India to draft a new health policy to ensure that the money allocated is spent as planned and as per the priorities and roadmap laid. So, the need for a National Health Policy became even more important (Delhi, 2002).

The overarching goal of the National Health Policy 2017 is *"the attainment of the highest level of health and well-being for all at all ages, through a preventive and promotive health care orientation in all developmental policies, and universal access to good quality healthcare services without anyone having to face financial hardships as a consequence"* (Ministry of Health & Family Welfare, Government of India, 2017).

"The primary aim of the National Health Policy 2017 is to inform, clarify, strengthen and prioritize the role of the Government in shaping health systems in all its dimensions- investments in health, organization of healthcare services, prevention of diseases and promotion of good health through cross-sectoral actions, access to technologies, developing human resources, encouraging medical pluralism, building a knowledge base, developing better financial protection strategies, strengthening regulation and health assurance" & further the National Health Policy 2017 would achieve the above-stated goals through *'Increasing access, improving quality and lowering the cost of healthcare delivery'* (Ministry of Health & Family Welfare, Government of India, 2017).

Research Background – Rationale

India has had three health policies so far, and India's policymaking has been at best ad hoc and despite setting the goals in each health policy, the policies failed to achieve the goals and shifted the goalposts. The health policy of 1982 mentioned about achieving 'Health for All' by 2000, and in the eight five-year plan the focus was changed to 'Health for the underprivileged'. Similar is the scenario with regards to other goals. In fact, *"NHP 2002 'does not claim to be a road-map for meeting all the health needs of the populace of the country"* (Gupta R. P., Healthcare Reforms in India: Making up for the lost decades, 2016, p. 260), and when a national health policy makes such a statement, it poses a serious question mark on the planners and implementors on the future health policies. If we look at the data of NFHS-5, and compare it to NFHS-4, the indicators for women's and children health have deteriorated over time than improving!

So, it is important to research into the policymaking process to help the health planners to make policies which don't repeat the mistakes of the past and address the issues in a holistic manner.

Scope of the Study

The study will have impact on planners for formulating a policymaking process addressing various components. Besides, it will be helpful to states considering formulating their state health policies. This study will help policy planners and policy makers use a structured process for inclusive and robust policymaking.

Purpose of the Study

The aim of present research is to study the health policy making process in India and make recommendations for developing a transparent and inclusive mechanism to improve policy-making process. To study the health policy process and its components such as (a) Agenda Building and Policymaking, (b) Planning, (c) Implementation, (d) Monitoring and Evaluation and (e) Identify the problems in each of these components, role of key actors involved in the process of policy making with regards to healthcare in India and suggest strategies to improve the health policy making process in India.

Research Questions

- What is the role and need for health policy in India?
- What has influenced the policies in health?
- What is the level of awareness regarding health policies among participants?
- Have the earlier policies achieved their goals?
- What are the challenges to formulate health policy in India?
- What are the problems and challenges in each of the identified components of Health policy 2017?
- What is the importance and involvement of key actors in the policy making process with regards to healthcare in India?
- How can we improve the health policymaking process in India?

Structure of the Study

The study covers the literature on policy, policy making process and its components, the administrative set up of healthcare in India, the national program - Ayushman Bharat and its mandate, various other national missions on health, challenges of healthcare policymaking, understand the policymaking process and make appropriate recommendations on each component of the policy making process.

The study makes recommendations on all four aspects of the policymaking process i.e., agenda setting and policy making, planning, implementation, and monitoring and evaluation with regards to awareness, communication, data, technology, capacity building, evidence-based research, and the health policies for states.

Policymaking

National health policymaking is a complex and dynamic process and varies from one country to another. *'The National health policies, strategies, and plans play an important role in defining a country's vision, priorities, budgetary decisions, and course of action to improve and maintain its people's health. Most countries have been developing national health policies, strategies, and plans for decades to give direction and coherence to their efforts to improve health'.* (WHO, 2017)

'The 'policy process' is often presented as a linear, rational process moving from formulation to implementation (Exworthy, 2008).

The formulation of health policies is complex process, and it depends on multiple scientific, economic, social, and political factors (Brownson, Chriqui, & Stamatakis, 2009).

The policy making process is undergoing a change everywhere. Earlier the policy analysis had a focus on government or public sector machinery which included politicians, bureaucrats, and interest groups. And over time, this has witnessed a shift as pointed by researchers in policy and policymaking. Now the stakeholders involved in the policy process are increasing and the new stakeholders include the private sector. Civil society organizations, also play a crucial role in defining the policies in healthcare. The public private partnerships had also impacted the policy formulation besides the global civil society. Technology is adding another dimension in being an influencer in policy (Walt, et al., 2008).

The Policy-Making Process (PMP) includes all aspects of how policies are initiated, formulated, or specified, organised, communicated, executed, and assessed. On reviewing the literature on the policymaking process, it gets clear that the area has remained largely theoretical, and the focus has been on important component, which is the agenda setting, and the initiation mechanisms for policy change, which can rightly be called as the 'triggering events'. When we consider the importance of the topic, the literature available is inadequate with regards to the empirical studies on the model of development of policies (policymaking process). The process/outcome model of policymaking will certainly include the following: initiation mechanisms, or triggering events, the agenda setting, politics, and the subsequent outcomes (intended vs. unintended) (Marchal, Arcens, Coates, & Brouwere, 2005).

The most well-known method to comprehend the PMP is adopting the stage heuristic method (Sabatier and Jenkins-Smith, 1993). This entails breaking down the approach method into steps while acknowledging that this is theoretical and does not accurately represent the reality. Nonetheless, it is critical to analyse policymaking as it encompasses the following stages:

1. *Problem Identification*: Examine how problems are included in the policy agenda and why some topics aren't discussed.

2. *Policy Formulation*: Examines who all are involved in policy formulation, how the approaches are discussed and decided, and then communicated between policymakers.
3. *Policy Implementation*: The most overlooked phase of policy development is the policy implementation, and is viewed as distinct from the first two steps. This step includes drafting the implementation framework with targets linked to programs for achieving the objectives as enshrined in the health policy.
4. *Policy Evaluation*: The verification of a policy's accomplishments, outcomes, or deficiencies. This distinguishes what happens once a strategy is implemented in terms of monitoring it, irrespective of whether it achieves its goals or has unforeseen consequences. At this stage, techniques are altered or discontinued, and new policies are implemented (Azline et al., 2018).

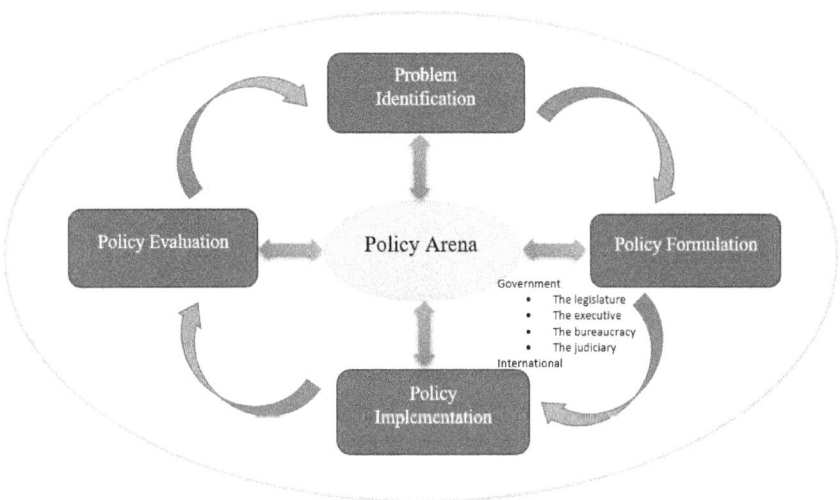

Figure 1: Policy Making Cycle (Reference: Azline et al., 2018)

Policy Arena

Policy arenas are platforms or the sites where the policymaking process happens or is conducted, including executives, legislatures, courts, semi-public entities, regulatory agencies, and expert committees. These stakeholders offer possibilities and certain limitations in policy creation and have specific norms for access, competency, information sharing, and decision-making which may have evolved over time (Timmermans, 2001). In a certain arena, there will be numerous players and actors with varied degree of influence and decision-making authority in a specific area (Azline, Abdullah, Iszaid, & Syahira, 2018).

The policy arena is divided into two parts: the government or state arena and the international arena. The several branches of authority within the government system, namely the administrative, legislative, and the judiciary are the state's stakeholders (Bulger RE et al., 1995). The administration branch makes decisions about national policies, and the bureaucracy refers to all systems and procedures about the implementation of policies. The legislative branch oversees adopting policies through the legislature, whereas the judicial branch oversees interpretation and enforcement of the policies (Bulger RE et al., 1995, Separation of Powers. Legislative, Executive, Judicial, 2018).

Various international organizations, international donor agencies, multi-lateral organizations, bi-lateral agreements, and the Sustainable Development Goals (SDGs) would fall under the international arena.

Decisions on Policy Changes

A policy shift is sometimes necessary to accommodate novel approaches, changing scenarios, beneficiaries, changing socio-economic conditions, and the policy changes may include measures such as implementing programs with new standards or changing criteria of existing programs. Policy changes entail a complex process. Policymakers consider multiple factors that influence their decision-making, including evidence of impact on health, priorities of stakeholders, feasibility, political and social considerations, and efforts of advocacy groups. Among these, evidence-based research to guide decisions taken to change the policies is an essential step in this complicated process (Tabak et al., 2015).

Attempting to learn from our own experiences and that of other countries is essential. Understanding the shortcomings of the earlier health policies would help us recognize the problems and strategize to develop a robust health care policy. We could also learn from the policies formulated by other neighbouring and developing countries such as Sri Lanka and Bhutan (Pillai RK, 2016).

Challenges

In India, it is difficult to establish health equity due to pervasive discrimination and avoidable inequities inherent in our system. Additionally, limited resources and knowledge adds to poor systemic preparation to handle the issues of inequality. Hence, health policy is essential to establish and maintain equitable health systems. Also, the bureaucracy runs the system, and if there is no clear and long-term policy, the programs depend on the personal disposition of the bureaucracy and change with the political regimes, and the same can lead to adhocism, so a national health policy is important for clarity, commitment, and continuity.

The important figures involved in policy planning (often exclusively), are development agencies, donors, the district administration, the state and national governments. Greatest challenge in PMP is the conflict of interest between various stakeholders and government, and their reluctance to adopt changes. The involvement of non-governmental or the civil society organisations in the planning process is minimal (Gopalan SS, 2011). This lack of integration impedes the development of a holistic and inclusive policy, resulting in inadequate healthcare delivery.

With regards to the Health Technology Assessment; In India, it was found that the policymakers at the lower levels don't have the desired knowledge on the subject (Jain, Hiligsmann, Mathew, & Evers, 2014). Similarly, public health specialists may be experts in their area of study but have very little understanding about the policy planning process and its implications. Individuals striving for health improvement, whether an educator, clinician, or a service provider, should understand the procedures for changing private and government sector policies to improve the health care system. Although researchers and policy experts have concrete information to improve the healthcare, but it is exposure and learning at the field level that offers a completely new perspective to the goal of enhancing and preserving people's health.

Therefore, it is mandatory to carry out stakeholder analysis and develop a strategy that can help in formulating an inclusive policy. Influence and power along with attitude and interest are important factors affecting formulation and execution of an effective public health policy. Evaluation of the extent of interest and support of stakeholders towards developing a policy should be performed using metrics including influence (low/high), power (low/medium/high), attitude/support (positive/neutral/negative) and interest (low/medium/high) (Franco-Trigo, L et al., 2020).

Once the desired stakeholders are identified, it will be possible to develop effective strategies and approaches to overcome the barriers in PMP as depicted in Table 1:

Table 1: Barriers and strategies to consider for effective PMP

Barrier	Strategies
Lack of value placed on public health or health care	Advocacy at all levels; that is, government, financial and technical institutions, private sector, communities, etc.
Insufficient evidence base	Identify and use evidence from different and authentic sources and promote research
Mismatched timelines	Communication and coordination between stakeholders and implementers
Power of vested interests	Build alliances in support of a policy to reduce power imbalance
Isolation of researchers and other necessary stakeholders	Raise awareness about need for inclusion to enrich and improve the process of policymaking
Lack of skills to influence evidence-based policy	Education on communication and the art of persuasion
Complexities of the policy-making process	Acceptance, understanding and persistence

Literature Review

Prioritizing Health

From Disease Capital to Death Capital, India's transition has been gradually building up due to lack of foresight and focus. Which is evident on the policies about health. Considering that 162 years ago (1859), the British Government had done a study on the issues that remain as glaring gaps for the healthcare policy and implementation. Even today, if we go beyond forty kilometres of any major metro town in India, the sanitary conditions and water supply are still the same, and for other category of towns, the scenario may be worse (Gupta R. P., Health Care Reforms in India: Making up for the Lost Decades, 2016, p. 90). With time, other factors like lifestyle have also added to this scenario worsening the already complex problem. The result is that India represents a significant portion of the world's illness burden, with 9.7 million deaths (1/5th of the total deaths occurring worldwide) and 486 million disability-adjusted life years (DALYs). Communicable diseases, maternal, perinatal, and nutritional disorders contributed to more than one third of the total national DALYs in India (Menon et al., 2020). The total estimated annual maternal deaths were 26,437 deaths in 2018 (Maternal health. UNICEF's concerted action to increase access to quality maternal health services, 2021). The child mortality rate in children below the age of five is 34.3 per 1000 live births as of 2019 (UNICEF Data: Monitoring the situation of children and women, 2021). Life expectancy for men at birth is 68 and for women is 71 as of 2019 (Life expectancy at birth-India, 2021). When we look at the above data, we see improvement in certain health indices such as child mortality and life expectancy within India while we are yet to improve maternal deaths and DALYS in the Indian population.

Health - Economic Growth and Development

A country aspiring to be developed needs quality human resources and therefore good health, and wellbeing is the important pillar for development of a country besides education and infrastructure. The reason why health becomes the most important pillar; as without health, one cannot realise the benefits of other pillars- education or infrastructure. Health plays an important role in country's economic development both directly and indirectly. The direct effect of health is visible in the labour productivity and the indirect one is the incentive effect. The link between health and labour productivity is that the greater the number of people in good health, the higher the country's economic growth. The incentive effect encompasses the effect of health on a person's life expectancy and a greater chance to invest in education and therefore contribute better to the labour market. Economic growth is directly related to the educated workforce in the country (Finlay, J., 2007). A ten percent increase in the survival rate of adults enhances the labour input per worker of 6.7 per cent and in terms of GDP per worker, it enhances by about 4.4 percent (Weil, 2005). The Growth Report (Commission on Growth and Development, 2008), makes a key recommendation to invest in nutrition, health, and cognitive development of children during the pre-school years. These initial investments could lead to person's lifelong earnings and health. The report further mentioned an example of a 35-year longitudinal study in Guatemala, it reported that men who were given protein supplement in the first two years earned an average wage 46 percent higher than men who consumed calorie-based supplement. So, investments in health lead to better productivity and higher income.

All over the world, it has become evident that the social sector, which includes education, health including the medical care, housing, sanitation, and water supply are crucial for the economy and country's growth. Improvement in the social sector directly affects agriculture, and industry sectors. Development of the social sector increases economic growth by means of it providing healthy, educated, and skilled workforce that demonstrates greater participation in developmental activities. Physical capital and labour force of a country increases and therefore increases the national income of the country. Better health enables the person to work, earn, and invest and this is a contributor to economic growth, which leads to greater domestic market opportunities, and international trade.

India's investment in the social sector is far behind the other BRICS nations (Brazil, Russia, India, China & South Africa) in social sector achievements as a result of the insufficient funding when it comes to the public investments on health and education, according to a study by the Associated Chambers of Commerce and Industry of India. Realizing that investments in the social sector will cause overall growth and development of the socioeconomic sector, the Government of India has devised several policies and programmes since independence, but the progress hasn't been noteworthy. In the 1968 policy, GoI planned to invest 6 percent of GDP into the education sector but the current spending on education is around 3.5 percent (Government expenditure on education, as a percent of GDP). The percentage GDP spent on healthcare is also in the same range, around 3.5 percent (Current health expenditure (percent of GDP) – India). This allocation of budgets on human development is grossly inadequate in India considering 75 years of independence (Mishra, P K and Mishra, S.K., 2015).

Health Indicators - National Family Health Survey (NFHS)

The National Family Health Survey 2015-2016

The NFHS 2015-16 reported the following observations:

1. Antenatal care among women (aged 15-49) increased from 80 percent in 2005-06 to 84 percent in 2015-16. Utilization of health care facilities for delivery increased significantly from 39 to 79 percent.
2. The under-five mortality rate and infant mortality rate were highest in rural areas.
3. For children who received all their basic vaccinations; there was 19 percent increase in the number of such children vaccinated (in the age group of 12-23 months).
4. The Aanganwadi service was utilized by only 54 percent children (under the age of 6), 54 percent pregnant women and 49 percent breastfeeding women.
5. As per recommendation, breast-feeding in the first hour of birth was followed in only 42 percent children. Stunted growth was reported in 38 percent children below the age of 5; 21 percent were wasted; 36 percent were underweight; and 2 percent were overweight. Undernourishment was observed in children born to illiterate mothers.
6. Number of households with at least one member covered by health insurance or under a health scheme were < 29 percent. Aadhar card was furnished by only 69 percent of the population.
7. HIV prevalence among men, decreased from 0.36 percent to 0.25 percent in the ten-year period from 2005-06 to 2015-16.
8. Anaemia in women and men aged 15-49 years was reported to be 53 percent and 23 percent respectively, and medically treated tuberculosis was reported in around 305 per 100,000 population (Tarun Gidwani. National Family Health Survey (NFHS-4) 2015-16: India, 2017).

Many of these public health outcomes are impacted by a range of social, economic, and political circumstances. It is vital to tackle structural issues, as some of these health inequalities may be due to unfair allocation of basic social goods, power, and resources (Narain JP,2016). Addressing these health inequalities should be considered as the key objective while forming public and healthcare systems policies, together with addressing the efficiency, exposure, and vulnerability to illness, while aiming to attain equality (Narain JP, 2016).

'Equity in healthcare' has been the guiding principle for decades for policy makers, in order to guarantee that the healthcare delivery is as per the needs of poor and the marginalised populations.

National Family Health Survey – 2019-21

The scope of the fifth round of the Survey (NFHS-5) was expanded to cover new topics like pre-school education, disability, access to toilets, death registration, bathing practices during menstruation, and abortion. The scope of this survey has been widened to include newer indicators like the waist and hip circumference, and the age band for blood pressure and blood glucose has been expanded. Usage of internet is a new addition and rightly so, given the important of technology driven care.

According to NFHS-5:

- 1020 is the Sex ratio of the total population (number of females per thousand males).
- 41 percent of the Households have a member covered under health insurance/ financing scheme.
- Women who have ever used an internet is 33 percent and for men, this number is 57.1 percent.
- Neonatal mortality rate per 1000 live births stands at 24.9.
- IMR stands at 35.2.
- Under-five mortality rate (U5MR) is 41.9.
- In the first trimester, 70 percent mothers had an antenatal check.
- 95.9 percent of the registered pregnant mothers have received a Mother and Child Protection (MCP) card.
- Average OOP (Out of Pocket) expenses for delivery in a public health facility stands at Rs.2916.
- 79.1 percent of the children received post-natal care from a doctor/ nurse /LHV/ANM/Mid-wife/ Other health personnel within 48 hours of delivery.

- 21.5 percent births were delivered through caesarean section in country. In the private health facilities, the percentage of births with caesarean section stands at 47.4 percent. Whereas, in the public health facilities, the births delivered through a caesarean section is 14.3 percent.
- percentage of children under the age of five who are stunted (height-for-age) stands at 35.5 whereas, 19.3 percent children under five years are wasted (weight-for-height).
- 7.7 percent of children under five years are severely wasted. This was 7.5 percent in the previous round of NFHS.
- 3.4 percent children under five years are overweight, which in the previous NFHS stood at 2.1 percent.
- Women with a high-risk waist-to-hip ratio (≥ 0.85) are 56.7 percent, and men with high-risk waist-to-hip ratio (≥ 0.90) are 47.7 percent.
- The percentage of children between the age group 6-59 months who are anaemic (< 11.0 g/dl) is 67.1, and in the earlier NFHS round this was 58.6 percent.
- The percentage of non-pregnant women between the age group 15-49 years who are anaemic (< 12.0 g/dl) is 57.2, and in the earlier NFHS round, this stood at 53.2 percent.
- Men between the age group 15-49 years who are anaemic (< 13.0 g/dl) is 25 percent, and in the earlier NFHS round this was 22.7 percent.
- This is the first time that NFHS has captured the blood sugar in adults (aged 15 years and above). The findings indicate that 6.1 percent women have high blood sugar level (141-160 mg/dl), 6.3 percent very high (> 160 mg/dl) and 13.5 percent high or very high (>140 mg/dl) or taking medicines to control blood sugar level. Amongst men, 7.3 percent men have high blood sugar level (141-160 mg/dl), 7.2 percent very high (> 160 mg/dl) and 15.6 percent high or very high (>140 mg/dl) or taking medicines to control blood sugar level.
- Hypertension amongst Women: 12.4 percent women aged 15 and above have mildly elevated blood pressure (Systolic 140-159 mm of Hg and / or Diastolic 90-99 mm of Hg). 5.2 percent women have moderately or severely elevated blood pressure (Systolic $\geq$ 160 mm of Hg and / or Diastolic $\geq$ 100 mm of Hg). 21.3 percent of women have elevated blood pressure (Systolic $\geq$ 140 mm of Hg and / or Diastolic $\geq$ 90 mm of Hg) or are under medication to control blood pressure.
- Hypertension amongst Men: 15.7 percent men aged 15 and above have mildly elevated blood pressure (Systolic 140-159 mm of Hg and / or Diastolic 90-99 mm of Hg). 5.7 percent men have moderately or severely elevated blood pressure (Systolic $\geq$ 160 mm of Hg and / or Diastolic $\geq$ 100 mm of Hg). 24.0 percent of men have elevated blood pressure (Systolic $\geq$

140 mm of Hg and / or Diastolic ≥ 90 mm of Hg) or under medication to control blood pressure.
- 1.9 percent women have ever undergone a cervical cancer screening, 0.9 percent for breast cancer and 0.9 percent for oral cancer.
- 1.2 percent men have ever undergone an oral cavity screening to detect oral cancer.
- 8.9 percent women aged 15 and above have used any form of tobacco and 38 percent men have used any form of tobacco.
- 1.3 percent women aged 15 and above have consumed alcohol and 18.8 percent men aged 15 and above have consumed alcohol.
- When it comes to the consumption of alcohol for both men and women, it is more in rural areas for women, 1.6 percent women have consumed alcohol in the rural area and 0.6 percent in urban areas and for men, this is 19.9 percent in rural areas and for urban areas, the figure is 16.5 percent.

(Ministry of Health & Family Welfare, Government of India, 2022).

If we compare the data from NFHS-5 with the earlier round (NFHS-4), there is a deterioration in the health of children, women and men when it comes to wasting, stunting, anaemia. This raises a red flag on the impact of policies on these issues and, the need for improving the policymaking process to ensure that the health improves over time due to the appropriate policy interventions.

Evolution of Health Planning and Policies

When the imperial rule in India came to an end, the people of India had hoped for a fundamental reform in the exploitative socio-economic system that the British had fostered and solidified. However, the hopes faded when it became clear that the new authorities were little more than activists from the old colonial regime.

Constitution of India & Health

Constitutional & legal mandate – The Right to Health!

Constitution is the ultimate reference point for legal rights and how the country is run through various institutions and laws. The planners and authors of the constitution realised the importance of health beyond the social and political significance. The constitution makers ensured that the Indian Constitution has clear provisions with regards to the right to health and well-being for the citizens. These are outlined in the Directive Principles of State Policy and Schedule 7 of the Indian constitution. But it is important to note that directive principles are non-justiciable under the Indian constitution.

Article 39(e), Article 39(f), Article 41, Article 42, and Article 47 have dealt with the subject of nutrition, education, standard of living, social security and working conditions amongst others to deal comprehensively with the issue of health for all ages. Specific references to health provisions have also been made in 7th Schedule under Article 246 of the Constitution.

The constitution of India made health a state subject but there are aspects of health that fall under the central and concurrent list, besides the states.

Central List

Item No. 28- Includes the port quarantine, which includes hospitals associated with, seamen's and marine hospitals.

Item No. 55 – deals with regards to the regulation of labour and safety in mines and oilfields.

State List

Item No. 6 – deals with the public health and sanitation, hospitals and dispensaries.

Item No. 9 – deals with the relief for the disabled and unemployable.

Concurrent List

Item No. 16 – includes lunacy and the mental deficiency, including places for the reception or treatment of lunatics and those with mental deficiencies.

Item No.18 – deals with the adulteration of foodstuffs and other goods.

Item No. 19 – deals with the drugs and poisons, subject to the provisions of entry 59 of List I with regards to opium.

Item No. 20A- deals with the population control and the family planning.

Item No. 23- deals with the social security and social insurance; the issue of employment and unemployment.

Item No. 24- deals with health conditions as it deals with the issues related to the welfare of labour including conditions of work, provident funds, employers' liability, workmen's compensation, invalidity and old age pensions and maternity benefits.

Item No. 25- deals with education, including technical education, medical education, and universities, subject to the provisions of entries 63, 64, 65 and 66 of List I.

Item No. 26- deals with legal, medical, and other professions.

Item No.30- includes vital statistics including registration of births and deaths.

Some scholars are of the view that the British did not give the desired importance to healthcare and so the authors of the constitution have attempted to fill this gap by stating that, the state shall regard its primary duty to the raise the nutrition status , the standard of living of the general populace and improve public health (Rameshwaram, 1989). (Gupta R. P., Healthcare Reforms in India: Making up for the lost decades, 2016, pp. 7-8). Despite the clear provisions about health in the constitution, healthcare policies were not framed in line with the constitution, and it took thirty-five years to frame the first health policy, and till then, the gap was filled presumably through the five-year plans.

There were a lot of radical ideas being implemented by the new government after independence, and it was even documented in the first Five Year Plan (FYP), and other publications for the sectors which drive the economy, but health remained in perennial neglect from a focus, priority, or policymaking point of view.

In the first Five Year Plan, the core task of preparation is described as follows: *"The problem is not one of merely re-channelling economic activity within the existing socioeconomic framework; that framework has itself to be remoulded so as to enable it to accommodate progressively those fundamental urges which express themselves in the demands for the right to work, the right to adequate income, the right to education and to a measure of insurance against old age, sickness and other disabilities. The Directive Principles of State Policy enunciated in Articles 36 to 51 of the constitution make it clear that for the attainment of these ends, ownership, and control of the material resources of the country should be so distributed as best to subserve the common good, and that the operation of the economic system should not result in the concentration of wealth and economic power in the hands of a few. It is in this larger perspective that the task of planning must be envisaged".* In contrast to the 1948 Industrial Policy Resolution, the Second Resolution of 1956 affirmed these directive principles and made recommendation for a policy framework, to help the parliament in achieving its general policy of adopting the socialist model as the overarching goal of the social and economic policy.

The 2nd Five-Year Plan laid emphasis on the model of growth and the structure of socioeconomic relations and stated that the model should be designed in such a way that they result in not just a noticeable rise in national incomes and employment but also lead to equitable distribution of incomes and wealth. The second FYP indicated that private wealth should not be the primary factor for choosing future directions of a project. It aimed for a steady decline in the concentration of incomes, wealth, and economic power. Without that, the advantages of economic development cannot accrue to the comparatively less privileged segments of the society (Duggal, R., 2001).

Post-colonial history, shows the fast erosion of these progressive ideas, aims, and decisions. The plans and programmes of the states have had little effect on the fair (equitable) allocation of resources. The policies and programmes have aided in the consolidation of disparities and continuation of underdevelopment (Duggal, R., 2001).

Following colonialism, private medical practice has emerged as Indian health sector's largest contributor, as a strategy to invest in the growing economy. To be explicit, the health sector developed in a way that was consistent with capitalism's overall economic agenda. Consequently, India's health policy cannot be separated from the country's economic and industrial strategy.

From 1947 till 1982, India did not have any official health policy. The different committees formed from time to time were the source of most of the inputs towards the creation of health programmes (Duggal, R., 2001).

In the immediate years post-independence, India was largely involved in aiding and supporting the private sector's capital accumulation process by committing major investment for capital goods manufacturing, growth in infrastructure, and financial services. Education and health were considered non-priority sectors. The focus was on industrial growth (Duggal, R., 2001).

Agriculture revenue goes towards building massive infrastructure for agricultural industry's growth. Investments are made towards agricultural research and education, farming, fisheries, dairy development, food marketing, forestry, storage, agriculture, finance, cooperatives, and refinancing organisations to increase agricultural production and other consumables, such as food grains, sugarcanes, oilseeds, cotton, jute, milk, fish, and eggs (Golechha, M., 2015).

During the fourth five-year plan, the Basic Needs Program was established to enhance rural infrastructure and offer support to small and marginal farmers, and rural development programs (formerly termed Community Development Programmes) witnessed great success. These initiatives, however, have not made a substantial impact on addressing rural poverty (Golechha, M., 2015).

Industry, power, transportation, and communication areas were disbursed more than 55 percent of the planned total resources. In an industrial economy, this is the foundational economic infrastructure. In an impoverished nation like India, the state felt that it was important to allocate finances to these areas of economy while neglecting the social which fall under public good (education, housing, health, and social welfare). Here, the state had a critical role to play (Golechha, M., 2015).

While the second five-year plan spoke about socialism, the greater engagement of the state in these fundamental economic sectors was important for the capital goods sector to thrive. The affluent Indian middle class lacked the financial wherewithal to build the basic and capital goods sector and required infrastructure, and hence, the government was not left with any other option but to offer the assistance. In addition, the banking industry was nationalised just before the fourth five-year plan began, and it developed rapidly under the state's support. In return, the private sector was able to further expand its hegemony by amassing huge financial resources

(Golechha, M., 2015). Excluding the petroleum industry (which has historically accounted for over 70 percent of public business earnings), the public sector industry has been experiencing net losses in the basic and capital goods sectors. The private manufacturing sector used majority of the public business output for the finished products, therefore the public sector continued to report losses. Given that, despite five decades of the institutionalized planning, three-quarters of the Indians still live below the poverty line, and that industrialization only created jobs in the organised sector for about 10 percent of the workforce, it's evident the decades of planning did not improve the lives of the marginalized population (Golechha, M., 2015).

Contradictorily, the five-year plans made pitiful contribution to social sectors, with less than a quarter of the plan's resources invested in the sector. Social services were divided into three primary categories: education, health, and water (Golechha, M., 2015).

Health care facilities were not up to acceptable standards and quality. Even the ambitious goals envisioned by the Sir Joseph Bhore Committee during the time of independence are still decades away from being met. Between the two world wars, most industrialised countries had health care coverage far superior to that in India. Majority of the country's rehabilitative health care services were catered to by the for-profit sector (about two-thirds), while the public sector provides the vast majority of preventive and promotion services (Golechha, M., 2015).

Healthcare Policies

Health policy interventions were formulated for providing quality health care services, secure people from financial risk by making healthcare affordable, while also dealing with inequities associated with the geographic and socio-economic status of a person (Selvaraj S. et al., 2021).

One of the earliest review of healthcare in India happened 162 year ago when in 1859, the Royal Commission on the 'Sanitary State of the Army in India', submitted its report on the underlying causes of high death rate amongst British soldiers in India , and it cited the following reasons : A) Inadequate sewerage B) Water supply C) Poor drainage D) Ill-ventilated and overcrowded barracks (Harrison, 1994, p. 61). So, the start in terms of policy planning in its most primitive form started in India with the Royal Commission Report in 1859.

In India, structured health care policy formulation and planning started before independence. In fact, the first comprehensive health care assessment and policy report created in India was in 1946, before independence. The report was titled, the Health Survey and Development Committee Report, often referred to as the Bhore Committee Report. The committee made proposal for a National Health Service to be implemented in India, which would ensure comprehensive coverage to the whole population for free, by a sophisticated state-run dedicated health care service (Duggal, R., 2001, India. Health Survey and Development Committee, 1946).

Post the Bhore Committee report, the country had a centralized planning and development strategy, and health policies and priorities were formulated as part of the "Five Year Plans". The first National Health Policy was released in 1983, and it reaffirmed the necessity for comprehensive universal healthcare (Delhi, N., 1983). It proposed decentralisation of the health system, greater community involvement and growth of private sector to lessen the load on public sector, as proposed by the Alma Ata statement. The second National Health Policy was released in 2002, this highlighted the investment and equity concerns (MoHFW, 2002). NHP – 2002 emphasized the need for more funding and an institutional restructuring of the national public health initiatives to ensure equity in healthcare. The Policy also focused on those diseases which were the drivers of the disease burden existing at that time – TB, Malaria and Blindness from the category of historical diseases; and HIV/AIDS from the category of 'newly emerging diseases'. National Health Policy 2002 put 'Equity' as its independent goal for which it would like to be assessed in future, and most importantly, the NHP 2002 admitted that it did not have a roadmap for solving all the health problems of the country (National Health Mission, n.d.). One is left thinking, that if a national sectoral policy coming almost after two decades (NHP 2002) makes a statement like, 'We don't claim to be a roadmap to finding solution to all the health problems faced by the country', then, it is all the more important to relook at the policymaking process, so as to ensure inclusive and responsive policies that can lay the roadmap for solving health problems of India.

In 2009, the Government passed the National Health Bill providing for a legislative framework for ensuring the right to health and the right to health care (The National Health Bill: Ministry of Health and Family Welfare, Government of India. 2009). However, considering India's institutional and implementation capacity, the execution of equitable policy continues to be difficult, even though it is a global community health concern and not a unique one for India (Pritchett, L., 2009, Gwatkin, D.R., 2000).

Administrative Set-up, Financing and Management of Healthcare in India

NITI Aayog

Earlier, the apex planning body was the Planning Commission, which was disbanded in 2014, and NITI Aayog came into existence vide resolution of the Union Cabinet on 1st January 2015, and it is the country's official policy think-tank, providing policy inputs. NITI Aayog is led by the Prime Minister as the Chairperson, and the Vice-Chairman is of Cabinet Rank. Besides drafting strategic and long-term policies and programmes for the states and the centre, The NITI Aayog also provides the technical advice to the Centre, States, and the Union Territories on a wide range of issues and across sectors. NITI Aayog acts as a platform for the Government of India to bring States to act together in national interest with the spirit of cooperative federalism.

The NITI Aayog has been instrumental in giving critical feedback to strengthen the Ayushman Bharat Scheme. It has conducted an extensive peer review of the various health benefit packages and recommended packages under the PMJAY scheme. The NITI Aayog also proposed measures to incentivize the enhancement in quality of healthcare services, such as the development of Standard Treatment Workflow and Health Benefits Package Costing.

Since 2017, NITI Aayog has been spearheading the Health Index initiative working with the health ministry, and with the technical assistance provided by the World Bank. This index ranks the performance of States and UTs on multiple indicators such as health outcomes, governance, and processes.

NITI Aayog has also reviewed and made recommendations on various policy documents, and it reviewed and made recommendations on the drafts of National Commission for Homoeopathy (NCH) Bill, 2018, Indian System of Medicine Bill, 2018, and National Commission for Yoga and Naturopathy Bill, 2018 (NITI Aayog).

Administrative set-up

The Ministry of Health and Family Welfare (MoHFW) at the centre is led by a minister holding a cabinet rank, and is generally assisted by either one or more Ministers of State. The ministry's administrative set up is headed by the bureaucrat who is a secretary rank official to the Government of India, and the secretary has a team of additional secretary rank officials and joint secretaries, amongst others. But the policy level decisions are limited to joint secretaries and above. Earlier, the Ministry of Health & Family Welfare had more departments, but over the past few years, the departments have been re-organized. The Department of AIDS Control has been merged with the Department of Health and Family Welfare to form the National AIDS Control Organization (NACO). The Department of AYUSH has been carved out as an independent ministry and renamed the Ministry of Ayurveda, Yoga and Naturopathy, Unani, Siddha, and Homeopathy (AYUSH), which focuses on the advancement of education and research in the systems of Ayurveda, Yoga and Naturopathy, Unani, Siddha, and Homoeopathy (Gupta R. P., Health Care Reforms in India: Making up for the Lost Decades, 2016) .

The Union Ministry of Health and Family Welfare has two departments, each of which is headed by a Secretary to the Government of India: The Directorate General of Health Services (DGHS) provides technical advice on all medical and public health issues and participates in the delivery of various health services (Ayushman Bharat - Health and Wellness Centre, 2019). The Department of Health Research and The Indian Council of Medical Research (ICMR), New Delhi, is India's apex body for the formulation, coordination, and promotion of medical research. This is led by the secretary rank official who is a clinician with experience in medical research. (Indian Council of Medical Research).

There are several organizations under the Ministry of Health and Family Welfare including National Health Authority (NHA), National Health Systems Resource Centre (NHSRC), National Institute of Health and Family Welfare (NIHFW), to name a few.

The National Health Authority was formed to replace the National Health Agency, to give full functional autonomy to fulfil the mandate. The newly formed National Health Authority (NHA) is the apex body in charge of implementing India's mega health insurance scheme, "Ayushman Bharat Pradhan Mantri Jan Arogya Yojana," and has been tasked with the designing of strategies, developing the required technological infrastructure, and implementing the National Digital Health Mission now renamed as Ayushman Bharat Digital Mission (ABDM) to create a National Digital Health Ecosystem as outlined in the National Health Policy 2017.

The National Health Systems Resource Centre (NHSRC) was established in 2007 with the mission of assisting in the policy and strategy and providing technical assistance and mobilization to states, and for capacity building for the Ministry of Health (National Health Systems Resource Centre).

The National Institute of Health and Family Welfare (NIHFW) is an autonomous organisation under the Ministry of Health and Family Welfare of the Government of India, serves as the key technical institute in addition to being the think tank for the promotion of programmes initiated by the ministry across the country (National Institute of Health and Family Welfare).

Besides the above, the Healthcare delivery in India is spread across various ministries and departments as mentioned below:

1. Ministry of Chemical & Fertilizers (Department of Pharmaceuticals) looks after the pharmaceuticals, that constitutes about 50 per cent of the OOP health care spending (National Commission on Macroeconomics and Health, 2005, p. 64).

2. Ministry of Labour and employment for unorganized labour. This ministry runs the ESIC hospitals.

3. Ministry of Women & Child Development that looks after the 'big budget' Integrated Child development scheme (ICDS).

4. Ministry of Defence that covers ex servicemen contributory health scheme (ECIIS).

5. Ministry of Water Resources.

6. Ministry of Rural Development.

7. Ministry of Railways (Railway hospitals).

8. Ministry of Social Justice and Empowerment (Ministry of Health & Family Welfare , Government of India, 2013, p. 80).

9. Ministry of Urban Development.

10. Ministry of Surface transport (NHAI).

11. Ministry of Tribal Affairs.

12. Ministry of AYUSH.

13. Department of Health Research.

14. Department of AIDS control.

15. Ministry of Agriculture.

16. Ministry of Information and broadcasting (DAVP is under this Ministry).

17. Ministry of Industry. The Salt commissioner's office is under the Ministry of industry and is responsible for monitoring, production, and distribution of iodised salt to the states and UTs.

18. Ministry of Commerce - Policies related to export and import.

19. Ministry of Finance – Insurance Regulatory and Development Authority (IRDA).

20. Coal Department (Ministry of Mines).

21. Port Hospitals (Ministry of Shipping).

22. Steel plants (Ministry of Steel).

23. Refineries (Ministry of Petroleum & Natural Gas).

24. Thermal Plants (Ministry of Power).

25. Bureau of Indian Standards (BIS) and consumer protection act are under Ministry of Consumer Affairs, Food and Public Distribution (Gupta R. P., Healthcare Reforms in India: Making up for the lost decades, 2016, pp. 104-5).

26. National Accreditation Board for Hospitals & Healthcare Providers (NABH) responsible for accreditation of hospitals and healthcare is under Quality Council of India, which falls under the Ministry of Commerce & Industry.

Structure of Healthcare System in India

According to the erstwhile planning commission of India, the healthcare system comprises of:
1. Three stages; primary, intermediate, and tertiary medical and paramedical institutions.
2. Doctors and paramedics training institutions to train required professionals and provide continuous education.
3. District, State and Central Program Managers.
4. Health management information system to collect, manage, analyse, and interpret (Institute of Applied Medicine and Research).

It is to be mentioned that the erstwhile Planning Commission has been replaced by the central government's think tank, NITI Aayog, led by the Prime Minister to advice on policy issues.

Ayushman Bharat Scheme

The structure of health care delivery under the Ayushman Bharat initiative has introduced novel and important interventions to include the preventive care, promotive care and ambulatory care services at primary, secondary and tertiary levels. This has two components: 1) The Health and Wellness Centres and 2) the Pradhan Mantri Jan Arogya Yojana (PM-JAY) (Ayushman Bharat - Health and Wellness Centre, 2019) (Figure 2). This component (PM-JAY) of Ayushman Bharat was formed with the objective of providing financial support to 40 percent of India's households, which fall below the poverty line, to make available secondary and tertiary care services to them (Ayushman Bharat - Health and Wellness Centre, 2019).

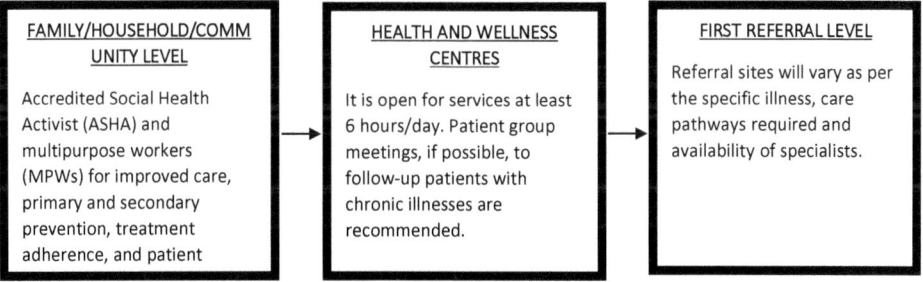

Figure 2: Structure of Health Care Delivery in India

(Reference: Ayushman Bharat - Health and Wellness Centre, 2019).

World's biggest health insurance scheme - PM-JAY is being implemented by the 'National Health Authority (NHA)'. The organization is under the Ministry of Health and Family Welfare and has full functional autonomy for delivering on its mandate.

The NHA has a Governing Board, which is led by the Union Minister for Health and Family Welfare. In terms of its organizational structure, NHA is led by the Chief Executive Officer, who holds a rank of the Secretary to the Government of India and is also the ex-officio member secretary of the governing board of the NHA.

NHA has its counterparts in every state through the State Health Agencies (SHAs), which operate on a society or a trust model. State Health Agencies also enjoy full operational autonomy like the national body for the roll out of the scheme at the state level.

Ayushman Bharat Digital Mission (ABDM) is being implemented by the National Health Authority by a multi-sectoral approach working with various ministries, the state governments, private sector and the not-for-profit CSOs.

The NHA has the overall functional responsibility for the implementation of the scheme, and this includes various functions like:

- Creating the documentation for the implementation of the scheme.
- Working to ensure that the scheme offering, and delivery is standardized and is interoperable.
- Define the pricing and premium and review it at regular intervals.
- Develop and ensure that there are checks and balances to ensure proper adherence to standard treatment guidelines.
- Ensure a system driven compliance to avoid frauds and misuse of the scheme.
- Look after the strategic purchasing from the private sector as per pre-defined norms.
- Set up a system to ensure timely payment to provider of healthcare services.
- Create a system for convergence of various schemes.
- Create a Digital Health Ecosystem with proper standards, interoperability frameworks in consultation with the other ministries.
- Work with insurance providers and IRDA for ensuring the success of PM-JAY.
- Carry out awareness programs for the scheme.
- Monitor the implementation of the scheme and make mid-course corrections based on the inputs received from time-to-time.

- Build strategic partnerships and collaborations with various stakeholders to further the objectives of the mission mode program and help in evidence-based policy making.

The National Health Authority has the responsibility for ensuring the organizational and technical support for the ABDM and to give the policy related inputs for the roll out of the mission and also, help in developing the self-financing model for the mission, coordinate with various stakeholders and solve the operational and technical issues that come during the implementation of the programme including the capacity building initiatives.

(National Health Authrority, 2021)

Health and Wellness Centres (HWCs)

As per the commitment of the National Health Policy 2017, in February 2018, the government announced the ambitious plan of converting all the existing 1,50,000 sub centres and primary health centres into Health and Wellness Centres (HWCs) to ensure comprehensive primary care, which includes, besides others, the maternal and child health services, management of non-communicable diseases, and free essential drugs and the diagnostic services. These HWCs were conceptualised to deliver universal and comprehensive primary health care services by catering to the marginalized population (Ayushman Bharat - Health and Wellness Centre, 2019).

Healthcare Financing

There is a rising need for sufficient funding to manage deficits in the finance required to set up quality health care delivery system in the country (Marten, 2014). Better communication between public policy makers and executives on healthcare expenditure would lead to a sustainable system covering the majority or all healthcare requirements of citizens. Policy changes impact countries, irrespective of their economic condition. Poor nations face problems to balance the cost of health care and its quality, while affluent countries allocate their resources towards managing the geriatric populations' health outcomes (Wang K.M., 2011, Jakovljevic M., et al., 2018).

India embodies an ominous paradox; its failure to provide to over 1.35 billion citizens with affordable health services, and yet being the 'pharmacy of the world' as the largest generic drug industry exporting affordable medicines to over 100 countries. It also has a booming private healthcare sector with a thriving medical tourism industry. The weak link in public infrastructure is drug unavailability, poor and dysfunctional laboratory equipment, severe scarcity of health care workforce, poorly financed public health systems (<1.04 percent of GDP), together with inadequate healthcare services delivery mechanism, which prevent a health care system from providing adequate and improved services (Golechha, M., 2015). The low level of investment in healthcare is a key factor that has led to poor health system functioning and poor health indices. This causes India to be burdened by a higher load of diseases resulting in households being trapped in poverty (Marten, R., 2014).

Indian leaders in politics and public health have attempted to develop and implement new programmes and best practices contributing to population health advances, As a result, more than 157,000 people have been engaged in the health care industry since the National Rural Health Mission was started in 2005 (Nair, H. and Panda, R., 2011). The infant mortality rate (IMR) declined from 68 to 28 for every 1,000 live births between 2000 and 2019 (Mortality rate, infant per 1,000 live births) – India, 2021). Janani Suraksha Yojana was able to ensure 88.50 percent institutional deliveries as of 2016. (Natalie Carvalho and Slawa Rokicki, 2019).

Financing public health is crucial for offering financial rights to the people for availing healthcare services thereby reducing OOPE. It is also important for ensuring better infrastructure, development of health workforce and provision of critical medications for free to the poor. Public health expenditure in India accounts for around 1.28 percent of GDP which is amongst the world's lowest. The country needs at least public health spending of 5 percent by 2025 to enable the healthcare delivery system to be accessible and efficient. It is also necessary to develop case management protocols and standard treatment guidelines, and outcome-based quality assurance standards (Srivastava, R.K. and Bachani, D., 2011, Chatterjee, P., 2014, Girvin, B., 2020).

Universal Health Coverage (UHC)

The UHC would ensure access to excellent, efficient, and affordable health care without imposing financial burdens on the people in need of healthcare services. Accessibility, availability, and affordability are the three main issues to be addressed in the healthcare delivery

(Planning Commission, 2011). The absence of these combined result in extremely high medical costs and Out-Of-Pocket (OOP) expenses. The government should ensure UHC to eliminate obstacles in the way of achieving good health and improve access to cost-effective and standard treatment. The UHC model should allow all residents to avail integrated health service package either through public health institutions or authorised private institutions for service deliveries such as diagnostics, medicines, vaccinations, or surgery without having to pay for utilizing the facilities and services (O'Connell, T., Rasanathan, K. and Chopra, M., 2014).

Foundation of the National Medical Service Corporation (NMSC)

Access to health care in India is best described by the 70:70 paradox; 70 percent of Indian medical costs are paid by individuals out of their wallets, of which 70 percent is exclusively used for medications and leads to poverty and debts. Every year, about 40 million Indians fall into poverty because of excessive OOP payments, and this number is before the COVID-19 hit us, and for sure, this number would have gone up drastically over the past two years.

Ensuring access to cheap essential medications is important to ensure the right to health and the universal health coverage tens of crores of Indians will have access to better care if the government has a mass procurement system, information technology driven, and online distribution system fronted by free distribution of generic medications to the public. Free provision of medicinal products through public institutions enables the public to improve their confidence in these systems. Already the states of Tamil Nadu and Rajasthan have centralised the procurement of medical supplies and have a decentralised logistics system, both of which have resulted in an increased access to essential medicines and in reducing the cost of medications (O'Connell, Rasanathan, & Chopra, 2014).

Further emphasis on evidence-based health policy and research on healthcare

Substantial improvement in community health results is undoubtedly driven by effective designing of healthcare research. Healthcare research efforts in India are not in sync with priorities in public health. In India, policies should be formulated by state-funded, research organizations as is done by the National Institutes of Health (NIH) as in the United States (O'Connell, T., 2014).

To enhance health outcomes, all significant health programmes and policies have to be carefully assessed. Research efforts need to be more interactive and designed to answer lacunae in health policies and programmes to formulate better health policies. The Government must focus on increasing research capability and capacity in research institutions to achieve this goal (Golechha M., 2014).

Human Resource for Health

India has a serious scarcity of professionals in the healthcare sector. Over 85 percent of the work force needs, that is, 75 percent of physicians, 80 percent of laboratory technicians, and 52 percent of auxiliary nurse midwife (ANM) positions in public health institutions across the country are vacant (Dandona, L., 2011). Though these figures may be old, as the number of medical institutions has increased and so has the medical and nursing colleges but still, the human resources are not available in rural healthcare settings as per the needs and with time, India's disease burden has also increased. Therefore, despite increased budget allocation, lack of human resources leads to failure of healthcare services and this needs to be attended to at the district level to strengthen the healthcare delivery.

Primary health strengthening: India has made progress in reducing the gaps between urban and rural, and the rich and the poor. Despite this progress, a large difference in the health care setup remains. It is still difficult to provide health care in the rural areas. Across the rural areas, only 69 percent of PHCs had at least one bed, and only 12 percent were maintained as per standards. These numbers are even worse in poorer states such as Bihar, where there is no sanitation and electricity. There is a serious problem of absenteeism of medical professionals in the rural areas (Banerjee A., 2020). Urban India has four-times more physicians and three-times higher the number of nurses than rural India (Nandan, D. and Agarwal, D., 2012).

Ayushman Bharat scheme by the government of India has established the political will to transform healthcare. To achieve and fasten progress, these policies need to be implemented as per the plan (Banerjee A., 2020). The government should also develop policies that improve health condition of urban poor people by implementing strategic methods that are effective, efficient, and outcome oriented. Reforms in line with the WHO health system strengthening framework should be implemented, and should include delivering services, employee health, information, medical goods and technology, funding, leadership, and management (Rao, K.D, et al., 2012).

Health Policy and Plans

India ran healthcare through its five-year plans and didn't have a comprehensive National Health Policy until 1983, when the government finally decided to draft its first health policy with a structured approach. There had previously been Five-Year Plans and suggestions from different committees which were used to create health initiatives. The health sector was part of the plans with clear objectives for each of the Five-Year Plans. Every plan featured several schemes, and each new plan added and removed a few schemes (Golechha, M., 2015).

During the mid-20th century, epidemic control was the primary goal of the health care system. The eradication of many diseases was thrust into high gear thanks to widespread public awareness efforts. Diseases like the malaria, smallpox, tuberculosis, leprosy, filaria, trachoma, and cholera were targeted by the different national campaigns, all of which used a technologically centred strategy. Each vertical programme included training the entire workforce. The National Malaria Eradication Program (NMEP) needed to train 150,000 personnel dispersed over 400 units for prevention of malaria and for the treatment aspects of malaria control (Golechha, M., 2015).

The strategy of launching massive campaigns was the idea borrowed from colonialists who believed in the modern system of medicine and that health could be improved by eliminating the germs that caused disease. However, societal factors such as poor diet, clothes, and shelter, and an unsuitable environment, are indeed the root causes of many illnesses. These concerns were not considered. To eliminate the illnesses, several national initiatives were put in place. The National Malaria Eradication Programme was established in the year 1953 with assistance from the United States Technical Cooperation Mission and technical guidance from the World Health Organization. Malaria was viewed as a global health issue at that time (Golechha, M., 2015).

One of the program's most critical initiatives was dichlorodiphenyltrichloroethane (DDT) spraying. The tuberculosis control programme included Bacilli Calmette-Guerin (BCG) vaccination, TB clinics, and home health care and follow-up. However, the focus was on vaccination with BCG, which served as a preventive measure. Similarly, to other areas of the economy, communicable illness policy was set by imperialist countries. Political and ideological sway came along with the financial assistance (Golechha, M., 2015).

Public health care delivery remained mostly unaltered over the first two Five Year Plans. More than three-fourths of medical care resources were allocated to cities, while rural regions got special attention as part of the Community Development Program (CDP). The past bears witness to the significance of this extra attention. CDP had already started to collapse even before the Second Five-Year Plan was implemented. The government has admitted to this failure (Golechha, M., 2015).

A primary healthcare unit (in a greatly diluted form from the Bhore Committee's proposal) was established under CDP for each development block, with a secondary health unit (which included a hospital along with a mobile dispensary) supporting each of the three primary health units. Improved environmental hygiene, particularly water supply provision and protection; appropriate disposal of animal and human wastes; addressing the control of epidemic illnesses like cholera, malaria, tuberculosis, smallpox, etc. was the goal of this healthcare unit (Golechha, M., 2015).

The medical treatment had no precedence in the structure of the health care organisation under CDP. Medical care facilities that provided mostly curative services (hospitals and dispensaries) flourished in urban areas (which grew independent of CDP). There was only one primary health unit (PHU) and one hospital for every 320,000 rural residents at the time of commencement of the third Five-year Plan (14 times fewer than the Bhore Committee proposed). In comparison, metropolitan regions had a hospital for every 36,000 population, and a hospital bed for every 440 people (Golechha, M., 2015).

The Mudaliar Committee was established in 1959 to assess the progress made after the first two 'Five-Year Plans', and to make recommendations for the future development of health care. For example, a study by the committee found that several highly contagious epidemic illnesses might be effectively controlled. Overall morbidity and mortality rates decreased, with deaths from malaria, cholera, and smallpox all being cut in half or drastically reduced. For the years 1956 to 1961, the mortality rate was down to 21.6 percent (Golechha, M., 2015).

The Mudaliar Committee also acknowledged that the basic health services were not yet available to half of the country. The Primary Health Care programme was undervalued from the beginning. End of 1961, there were only 2800 PHCs left. Despite the "irreducible minimum staff" proposed by the Bhore Committee, majority of the Primary Health Centres had insufficient human resources, with a large number of these PHCs being managed by ANMs or the public health nurses. The reality was that after completing their studies at public universities, the physicians were going into private practice. First and foremost, in the first two 'Five Year Plans', the focus was on specific communicable disease programmes. Yet only little assistance was offered to primary health facilities, where improvement was expected (Mudaliar Committee. 1962)

Rural communities rarely had accessibility to the government run programmes. The ground reality of the secondary and district hospitals was no better than the primary care centres. According to the findings, metropolitan regions have the bulk of infrastructure (Mudaliar Committee. 1962).

The Committee proposed that instead of expanding PHC, district hospitals should be equipped with mobile clinics to treat patients who do not have health insurance. This would be done in stages, starting with an immediate upgrade of PHC facilities. However, to satisfy the rising need for medical treatment, the urban health infrastructure was expanded, with money provided by the state government. Planning Commission investments went into preventive and promotional initiatives, while state governments focused on curative care (Mudaliar Committee. 1962).

Regarding medical personnel resources, the Mudaliar Committee recommended efforts to enhance doctor and other staff services in rural regions to entice doctors and staffs to rural regions (Mudaliar Committee. 1962).

The committee mentions that, aside from the considerable enhancement in the number of physicians, the availability of associated health workers remained woefully inadequate. Therefore, the committee urged that the medical education should be allocated a significant portion of public health expenditures to fill the need gap (Batliwala S. 1978).

The Mudaliar Committee examined the health system for a decade and found many trends and shortcomings, but the Committee remained optimistic that medical care could be improved and that large additions to the medical workforce might help improve the country's community health. A larger budget was allocated towards educating doctors in particular specialties. This resulted in the dramatic rise in medical school seats, which more than doubled in just one planning year. The number of nurses and other support staff hired remained unchanged (Batliwala S. 1978).

A third Five Year Plan began in 1961, and this plan addressed issues including lack of health workers, delay in the construction of the PHC buildings and the staff quarters, and the insufficient training facilities for the various kinds of healthcare workers needed in the rural regions. The third Five-Year Plan mentioned about the lack of adequate health care facilities, physicians, and other medical staff in rural regions as one of the key failings of previous Five-Year Plan. The doctor-syndrome preoccupied planners, and a rise in the availability of health human resources meant more physicians rather than other health workers. While this third plan acknowledged the need for more support staff, no concrete measures were outlined towards achieving this objective. Lack of funds remained a continuous barrier to training and establishment of support staff. While this may be true, the proposed expenditures for new medical institutes, the setting of the preventive and social medicine, the department of psychiatry, completion of the AIIMS, and schemes to upgrade medical college departments for postgraduate training and research have all remained high. The third plan seriously considered suggesting a pragmatic idea to address the long-standing issue of the shortfall of doctors in the rural areas, mentioning, "that an animated course for the training of medical support staff should be initiated and after completion of their five years at a PHC they could finish their education to become full-fledged doctors and continue in public service".

This plan era saw a rise in PHC numbers despite the Mudaliar Committee's advice against it, although their health was the same as it had been in the second plan period. There was an influx of people working on the disease programme since it was vertically organised that way. Specially trained health professionals continued to offer services as per the recommendations made in 1963 by the Chadha Committee and it was implemented in the form of two multifunctional workers for every 10,000 people in the population at the time (Batliwala S. 1978).

When India implemented a government-sponsored family planning programme in 1951, it became the world's first country to attempt such a programme. In the first two plans, the Family planning (FP) programme was mostly conducted by non-profit groups under the auspices of

Family Planning Association of India (FPAI). In the third plan with growing birth and mortality rate, it was mentioned, "the objective of stabilizing the growth of population over a reasonable period must therefore be at the very centre of planned development". Thus, population control became obligatory. Under the programme, the camp method was put to test, and the government departments started to actively participate in the efforts for population control. In addition, Ministry of Health created a separate department for family planning (Chadha Committee, 1963).

Industrialised nations, and in particular, the USA had a strong effect on the significant emphasis on population management. A U.N. advising mission to India in 1966 strongly urged that health and family planning should be exempted from government regulations and should include policies to address nourishment and the health of the mother and child (Chadha Committee, 1963). This marked a turning point in India's health care system policy. This policy shift was necessary and despite its own internal pressures, was made possible due to the involvement of external entities approving this plan of action. A special committee was appointed for financial management and implementation of the family planning department plans (Banerji, D., 1973). The Chadha committee figured that the sterilization camp method had failed to achieve the objectives of the family planning programme and that the introduction of intra-uterine contraceptive device (IUCD) or a coil was a better idea. This committee also proposed the adoption of fixing targets, with rewards and incentives to motivate and incentivize. It proposed restructuring the Family Planning programme from horizontal to a vertical one, as in the case of malaria, and the inclusion of an additional health visitor for each PHC, to particularly oversee the ANMs for the program's target population. This Committee also proposed that private practitioners be retained at a cost of rupees hundred per hour for six hours of labour per week, with payment of rupee ten for every sterilisation and rupee two per IUCD insertion (Duggal, R., 2001).

The fourth five-year plan, which began in 1969, followed a similar path as the third plan, and drew heavily from the FYP II for information about the socialist social structure (FYP IV, 1969, 1-4) but the policies it pursued, plans and choices made during the meeting did not represent socialism. It doesn't mention the turmoil in society, politics, and the economy that occurred throughout the planned holiday time (1966-1969). In fact, the three years of instability had resulted in major adjustments to economic policy. But the fourth plan was entirely ignored. It bemoaned the lack of progress achieved in the PHC programme and reiterated the necessity for its strengthening. It urged for the creation of efficient machinery to expedite the construction of structures and the enhancement of the performance of PHCs via the provision of personnel, equipment, and other resources (Duggal, R., 2001).

It was the first time that PHCs had their own budget allocation. In addition to strengthening the foundation of the primary health centres, the sub-divisional and the district hospitals, which would serve as the referral hubs for Primary Health Centres, were emphasised. To strengthen the communicable diseases program, the significance of primary health care clinics was elucidated. Because of the spike in malaria incidence from 100,000 cases per year between 1963 and 1965 to 149,102 cases in 1966, the whole epidemiological trend was reversed (Duggal, R., 2001).

Although infant mortality rates had decreased and life expectancy had increased during the fifth Plan, the government acknowledged regretfully that health care facilities in rural areas, including hospitals, functionaries, beds, and health facilities were still insufficient despite these advances (Duggal, R., 2001).

This demonstrates that the government was aware of the growing urban health sector at the expense of the rural healthcare delivery. This was evident in the 5th FYP objectives, which are as mentioned below:

1) To increase the availability of healthcare services in rural areas under the Minimum Needs Programme (MNP) and addressing disparities in the healthcare delivery.
2) Improvements in district and sub-division hospital referral services.
3) Increased efforts to combat and eradicate communicable illnesses.
4) Enhance the quality of education and training.
5) Improvement in referral services in remote regions by making experts available to treat common illnesses.

To attain these objectives, techniques included the MNP, the Multipurpose Workers (MPW) training programme and providing special care to underserved and indigenous regions.

There have been significant advancements in health policy and delivery methods. Reforming health programmes aimed to build on previous successes in areas such as communicable illnesses, medical education, and rural infrastructure supply, among others. This was envisioned by the MNP, which said that it would be prioritized and be the first charge on developing outlays within the health sector.

As part of this proposal, health care workers were particularly educated as multipurpose health assistants, who would then be able to provide services to the public (Duggal, R., 2001).

When the Kartar Singh Committee was formed in 1973, it advocated for expanding the job responsibilities of workers like ANMs to train them in various functions. It was suggested that two such workers should serve population between 10,000 to 12,000. Hence, the programme of having multipurpose workers was initiated, aimed at retraining the existing cadre of vertical programme, and the different vertical programmes to be integrated in the main health care package for rural areas (Mukherjee Committee, 1966).

In 1977, the creation of a group of village-based health auxiliaries known as community health workers was established as another significant health strategy breakthrough. These part-time employees were chosen by the village and educated for three months in simple promotional and curative skills in allopathy and other indigenous medicine systems. MPWs were to oversee them, and the initiative was launched in 777 PHCs that already had MPWs on staff (Mukherjee Committee, 1966).

An important proposal of the Shrivastava Committee on the medical education and support personnel was accepted which resulted in the community health worker's programme. The committee proposed addressing rural areas' shortage of skilled workers. The committee stated, "the over-prominence on provision of health care through professional personnel under state supervision has been counterproductive." On one side, it devalues and destroys the old practice of having part-time workers, which the society used to teach and not utilize them, and proposed, with some modifications, part-time workers can continue to provide the base to establish a national health care programme. On the other hand, the overall quality of new professional services offered under state supervision were inadequate. This committee's extremely straightforward remark on the need to re-examine medical education and its associated components was significant since it shows that the money spent on health care was not reaching the intended beneficiaries – the end user. The committee's major suggestion was to have part-time health workers from the communities they have to serve and act as a liaison between them and the Multipurpose Workers (MPW) at the sub-centres (Mukherjee Committee, 1966).

The committee demanded a halt to the creation of new medical schools when it came to medical education. The committee stressed that expecting doctors to travel to rural regions was a mistake due to a variety of socioeconomic factors. This left them with only one choice for rural areas, the Community Health Workers (CHW) programme. This stance was backed with the historical notion that the problems associated with healthcare were quite different across the rural and urban populations, with the urban residents needing curative treatment and rural residents needing preventive. This is also discriminatory, as this paradigm imposes hardships on rural residents. Devolving of medical care began in 1967 with the Jain Committee Report, which looked at the medical care services, and advocated improving primary health care at the block and taluka level facilities, besides the district hospital infrastructure. The Jain Committee also proposed district-level unification of medical and health services under the Civil Surgeon/Chief Medical Officer. However, Jain Committee's proposals were the first to investigate medical care since independence and the first to talk about improving curative facilities in rural regions, but the recommendations were not taken seriously (Singh, K., 1973).

A situation of national emergency was declared during the fifth Plan (1975-77) and population control under the family planning programme was ramped up with coercion and violence being the strategy for the family planning programme.

Two things shaped the sixth 'Five Year Plan' (1980); the Alma Ata Declaration of 'Health for all by 2000 AD' (WHO), and the ICSSR-ICMR report. The strategy acknowledged the widespread discontent with the current medical and health care paradigm, which placed a premium on hospitals, specialty care and super specialization, and highly trained doctors, all of which are available primarily to the wealthy, and because which, rural areas and impoverished people are denied access to quality healthcare and medical services. The focus of the strategy was on establishing a community centric health care system. The strategies included the following:

a) The focus of the strategy was on establishing a health care system centred in the community. Priority should be accorded to health services in rural areas.
b) To train a significant number of community-based first-level health care workers under the supervision of MPWs and PHC medical officers.

c) Not to build more curative care infrastructure in metropolitan areas; and this would be authorised only in rare situations.

The strategy accorded importance for the need to link all connected programmes horizontally and vertically, such as the water supply, environmental sanitation, hygiene, nutrition, education, family planning, and MCH. As a result, it was decided that by 1995, the net reproduction rate should be equal to 1.

The first National Health Policy of India (NHP) came in 1983 and it suggested "universal, comprehensive primary health care services responsive to genuine community needs and priorities at a cost people can pay (MoHFW, 1983). The government's discussion of universal comprehensive health care after the Bhore Committee in the 40's was a positive step towards the goal of providing universal health care.

A policy statement is fundamentally representative of the views of those in power to define what they believe to be people's will. For a variety of reasons and circumstances, rulers and the ruled may not always agree. The implementation of a policy needs political will, particularly if it intends to dramatically alter the current situation. Whether or not political intent is translated into action is a function of both voter conscientization and the social concerns of those in government. The key features of the 1983 health policy are as presented in Table 2.

Table 2: Key points of the 1983 Health Policy

NHP-1983 Criticized the western medicine based curative cure approach
NHP-1983 laid special emphasis on comprehensive primary care, which included; preventive, promotive and rehabilitative health care
NHP-1983 emphasized decentralised system for health care, which would be low cost based on volunteers and paramedics and resting on the pillar of community participation.
NHP-1983 called for more prominent role for the private sector in healthcare delivery to reduce the burden on the government.
NHP-1983 called for a review of the existing legislative framework for a comprehensive and unified legislation for the nation.
NHP-1983 defined targets for achievement that were primarily demographic in nature
NHP-1983 aimed to deliver 'Health for all by Year 2000', and focussed on provision of integrated and comprehensive primary healthcare for all, adopting an inter-sectoral approach
NHP-1983 recommended the formulation of National Population Policy
NHP-1983 recommended the involvement of Volunteer Groups and NGOs
According to the NHP-1983, in medical research, besides focussing on the basic and fundamental research, higher priority must be accorded to the applied and operational research, including action research aimed at reducing the cost of healthcare delivery and achieving self-sufficiency in healthcare for the future. Top priority to be given to research on nutrition and to improving the health status of the community. Overall goal was a balanced development across basic, clinical, and problem-oriented operational research.

In the decade that followed the NHP in 1983, rural health care got special attention, and a large development effort for the primary health care facilities were conducted in the 6th and 7th Five-Year Plans to target one primary health centre for every thirty thousand population and one sub-centre for every five thousand of population. This goal has largely been achieved; but a few states failed to achieve this. Numerous studies on the rural primary health care have revealed that, despite availability of hard infrastructure, they are underutilised due to poor equipment, lack of efficient person-hours, inadequate supplies, inadequate doctors, faulty planning of various programmes, and the inadequate monitoring and evaluation mechanisms. This method was based on the idea of a health team, but it didn't function due to mismatch between training and job that was assigned to health professionals, inadequate transportation, and a lack of acceptable housing for the health team. Deprofessionalization, decentralization, and other tasks outlined in the 1983 health strategy, had taken place in a limited setting, but without community involvement. As shown by their healthcare seeking behaviour, the primary health care model being implemented in rural regions was never acceptable to people. Rural residents continue to use private health care, and they prefer the urban hospital for primary care when they do use public facilities (Shrivastava Committee, 1975, Nandraj, S. and Duggal, R., 1996, Kannan, K.P., et al., 1991, NCAER. 1991).

Regarding the NHP's objectives, only death rate and lifespan were a part of their plan. Fertility and immunization objectives did not reach expectations (despite the efforts and resources devoted to these programmes over the previous two decades that had targets connected to national disease programmes). There is mounting evidence of the growth of private sector in healthcare delivery since the national health policy, but states still deny adequate curative services to rural areas while supporting curative services in urban areas, and population control is still a priority programme (as recognised by the WHO).

As per the seventh Five-Year Plan, evolution of specialties and super-specialties should be pursued in a focussed approach to ensure regional distribution and the training across the super specialties would be encouraged in both the public and the private sectors. The spotlight on specific diseases like, AIDS, cancer, and coronary heart disease, and the expansion in the diagnostic business and corporate hospitals, demonstrate where the health sector's interests lie.

There was a severe economic downturn prior to the implementation of the Eighth FYP. The timeline for the FYP was accelerated by two years. However, despite this, the strategy remained unchanged. The eighth plan changed its motto to stress on health for the underprivileged rather than adhering to the goal of health for all by 2000 AD set in the national health policy 1983.

Parallel to this, it continued to promote privatisation by saying that, "private hospitals and clinics will be encouraged subject to maintaining basic standards and sufficient returns for the tax incentives", and this was in accordance with the new government policy. One of the criticisms of the NHP is its failure to give a push to public health infrastructure, thereby making it challenging for the common man to avail healthcare in public healthcare facilities (Ghosh, 2001).

However, the ninth 'Five-Year Plan' gives a thorough assessment of all initiatives and attempts to build upon the past successes going forward. The ninth plan included several ground-breaking concepts. It was encouraging to see references to the Bhore Committee report once again, putting the prevailing situation at that point in time in context with the Bhore committee's recommendations. One of the most significant goals of the Basic Minimum Services programme in the 9th FYP was to consolidate PHCs and sub-centres and ensure that the conditions for their successful operation were available. It was not easy to find physicians for PHCs and CHCs and therefore the plan proposed leveraging the local competent private practitioners by engaging them on part-time employment basis and/or renting out the PHC or CHC facilities for after-hours practice. Another suggestion was to create mechanisms to make referral services more effective.

The Education Commission for Health Sciences was established under the eighth 'Five-Year Plan', and some states had gone ahead and even established the University for Health Sciences in accordance with the 1987 Bajaj committee report recommendations. With these efforts, all health sciences were integrated, continuing medical education was enabled, and the quality of medical and health education improved. The ninth 'Five-Year Plan' included provisions to hasten this procedure.

A committee to examine public health was established during the eight-plan period. The group was known as the Expert Committee on Public Health Systems. According to the committee's findings, most communicable illnesses were on the rise again, and disease surveillance in the country had to be significantly improved. According to the ninth plan, districts were supposed to have a robust detection and response mechanism to quickly limit any epidemics that may develop. The committee's suggestions served as a foundation for the ninth five-year plan's health sector strategy, which aimed to reinvigorate the country's public health system to meet the country's changing health care demands. Additionally, the plan recommended the horizontal integration of all vertical programmes from the district level to improve the program efficiency and enable allocative decisions. The National Population Policy and the Family Planning Program were also reviewed under the ninth FYP. The program for the maternal and child health care were at the heart of this initiative, according to the Bhore Committee study. Assuring prenatal care, safe delivery, and vaccination were essential to lower new-born and maternal mortality, and this had an impact on contraceptive usage and fertility rates. The same rationale was adopted by the family planning programme, except that in the past they focused on sterilization. ANMs were first employed in the early 1960s specifically for the MCH programme, but the family planning programme took over at the field level. This programme continued throughout the 1970s and 1980s. MCH was renamed Safe Motherhood, and the enlarged immunization program was renamed the Universal Immunization Program. This program was merged with the ongoing Child Survival and Safe Motherhood (CSSM) program in the seventh five-year plan, although family planning remained the primary focus. CSSM, on the other side, was taken seriously since the eighth plan and into the ninth plan, and it later transformed into the RCH programme, which was based on the International Conference on Population and Development (ICPD)- The Cairo agenda, and this received external funding support to provide high quality integrated reproductive and child health care based on the demand. During this time, the National Population Policy was unveiled in a big way in the middle of the year 2000. Although it was an improvement over its predecessors, the fundamental goal was still population control and not population welfare. The primary issue was keeping track of the population; therefore, the objectives were also strictly demographic in nature.

National Health Policy 2002

India's track record for health policies was never planned or structured. Despite Bhore Committee recommending a health policy, the first policy had come only after 37 years in 1983. Later, almost nearing two decades since the NHP-1983, the need for a new health policy was felt because of changes in the healthcare landscape. Moreover, NHP-1983 had a mixed bag when it came to achievements, and of course, the lofty goal of 'health for all' was still a pipe dream. The objectives of the NHP 2002 was to *'achieve an acceptable standard of good health amongst the general population of the country'* (National Health Policy, 2002, p. 21);by decentralization, infrastructure upgradation & development, equitable access, increased investment from the central government, enhancing the role of private sector, preventive and curative care at the primary health level, integration of traditional system of medicine and rational use of allopathic drugs.

Key observations, references, and recommendations of NHP 2002:

- *It highlighted the success stories of the NHP 1983 like the establishment of primary healthcare centres, health volunteers, referral system, speciality and super speciality services, to encourage private investments, eradication of Smallpox and Guinea Worm disease & substantial drop in TFR & IMR.*

- *Noted that several complementary initiatives in the developmental sector, besides health, led to the improvement in health indicators. Still, the morbidity or mortality levels were unacceptably high.*

- *There has been resurgence in malaria during 1990's. Also, there has not been a significant decline in T.B. and the emergence of drug resistant T.B. has been a challenge, emergence of HIV/AIDS, the common water borne infections continue & the increase in life-style diseases coupled with the improvement in life expectancy had led to increased need for geriatric care services. Trauma care continues to be a significant burden.*

- *Challenge of addressing nutrition related issues especially among vulnerable sections.*

- *Lack of financial and administrative capacity led to the failure of 'Health for All by the year 2000'. New policy would expect to be formulated for achieving of public health goals taking into account the socio-economic conditions of the country.*

- *Public investment into health has declined from 1.3 percent in 1990 to 0.9 percent in 1999. 83 percent is out of pocket (OOP) spending. Investment from the centre has been stagnant but from the states, it has reduced from the earlier levels of 7 percent to 5.5 percent. Current per capita health expenditure stands at about Rs. 200, and that quality of public health services is sub-standard. There is a need for increased spending from the centre on health. NHP 2002 aimed at increasing the expenditure in health sector to 6 percent of GDP. It further aimed to apportion 2 percent of the GDP for public health to be achieved by 2010. Health being a state subject, it was expected that the state governments would increase their investment in health to 7 percent of their budget by 2005 and 8 percent by 2010. Central government would increase its contribution from the current 15 percent to 25 percent by 2010.*

- *Not only are the national averages with regards to health indices unacceptably low, but large gaps exist across the country with regards to health facilities leading to inequities and rural – urban divide, particularly for the vulnerable sections of the society. NHP 2002 recommended a change in the overall fund allocations towards the health sector and of the total allocations to health, 55 percent would be invested for primary health, 35 percent for secondary care, and 10 percent would be for tertiary care.*
- *Centre will continue to design the broad-based public health initiatives and states to have flexibility in implementation and NHP 2002 would address the role of centre and the states*
- *For public health programmes which lack a vertical structure, there is no separate delivery system at all and NHP 2002 envisioned reorientation and integration of all the existing national health programmes under a single field administration, barring a few major diseases till the prevalence is reduced. The NHP 2002 envisioned a separation of the role for monitoring and implementation. The state's role would be limited to overall monitoring of the targets, and implementation would be with autonomous bodies at the state and district levels with the involvement of elected officials, social activists, and government officials to facilitate informed decision making. Also recommended capacity development within the states for designing of public health projects for the local population and expected that public health administrators will need a mindset change and the staff at rural centres will need to be trained and reoriented to design appropriate intervention through the programmes and effectively implement them.*
- *Expressed dissatisfaction with regards to the public health facilities stating that less than one out of five people seek OPD and less than 45 percent seek the indoor treatment (IPD) avail from the dysfunctional public facilities. Even though most of the patients lack the financial means for private sector facilities. NHP recognised that distribution of medicines through the primary care was essential and recommended providing essential drugs through the primary health system funded by the centre, more frequent in-service training of medical and paramedical professionals, improving of primary care and levying of reasonable user charges for some secondary and tertiary care services for those who can afford to pay.*
- *Deputing medical personnel in rural areas has been a losing battle and to use the services of nurses, paramedics etc after imparting training must be explored along with*

easing out recruitment procedures and contractual employment, besides a mandatory two-year service in rural areas before awarding the graduate degree.

- *Deploying practitioners of indigenous system of medicines to extend the reach of health services. Also, the NHP dwelled on building credibility for the alternative systems. However, it stated that the policy on the alternative systems of medicine would be developed separately.*
- *The policy recommended an Increasing role of local self-government in delivery of health services in line with its objective of decentralizing healthcare delivery and urged the state governments to consider handing over of the programme implementation to the local self-government institutions by 2005.*
- *Doctors and nurses fall short of the norms needed for adhering to the minimal standards of patient care and NHP stated that minimum statutory norms for deployment of doctors and nurses in medical institutions should be introduced on an urgent basis, and it should be progressively reviewed and made more stringent.*
- *Educational facilities are unevenly spread, quality of education is highly uneven and sub-standard & syllabus is excessively theoretical. NHP suggested the setting up of the Medical Grants Commission for financing the establishment of the new medical colleges all over the country and upgrade the infrastructure of the existing institutions, development of need-based, skill-oriented curriculum with more practical training and focus on capacity building for the geriatric disorders and cutting-edge disciplines of contemporary medical research. Also recommended an increase in seats for postgraduates.*
- *NHP talked about ensuring the availability of public health professionals & the family medicine specialization and recommended that the seats be increased to achieve a goal where 25 percent of the seats are reserved for public health and family medicine courses. Public health specialization be encouraged for non-medicos as well.*
- *With regards to the issue of acute shortage of nursing professionals, the NHP recommended increasing the skill level of the nurses, setting up of training facilities for nurses subsidized by the central government. Also, it felt that there was a need for starting specialised training courses for super speciality nurses in tertiary care.*
- *On the issues of future health security of the country with regards to use of generics and vaccines, the NHP emphasized the usage of generics for essential medicines in public and private sector, resorting to fiscal disincentives for implementing the same in private*

sector and periodic review of the essential drug list. Also, more than half of the vaccines needed should be sourced from public sector.

- With regards to issue of healthcare in urban areas which are unserved and lack the basic standard of health care facilities, the NHP recommended the setting up of a proper urban primary healthcare structure with primary care as the first tier covering one lac population having an OPD and providing essential medicines, and a second tier being taken care at the government hospital. Financing for the same be met by the local self-government, state, and the centre. NHP also envisions the setting up of the fully equipped trauma care services in large urban agglomerations on hub and a spoke model.

- With regards to mental health, NHP envisioned a network of decentralised mental health services and upgrading existing physical infrastructure for Indoor treatments funded by the centre.

- NHP talked about the IEC strategy for improving awareness and for using it as a tool for behavioural change in the general population and target schools with priority in the new policy, and associate PRIs, NGOs and trusts with specific targets.

- On the issue of health research, the NHP expected an increase in the government funding to 1 percent of the total health spending by the year 2005 raising it to 2 percent by 2010. Focus of research would be newer therapeutic drugs and vaccines for tropical diseases, and HIV/AIDS on a mission mode basis. Private entrepreneurship will be encouraged in medical research.

- Role of private sector. NHP observed that private sector contributed immensely to the secondary and some tertiary care but the perception about the quality is that it is highly uneven, substandard, financially exploitative, and professional ethics is an exception. Regulation of private sector has become imperative, with standards, for medical and health practice. NHP welcomed the private sector participation at all levels of healthcare delivery. According to the policy, the private sector was expected to play a significant role in primary and tertiary sector and moderate in secondary care in the urban areas. NHP envisaged setting up the necessary regulation for minimum standards for clinical and medical institutions by 2003. Starting with statutory guidelines and moving to accreditation for clinical practice and delivery of medical services, setting up private insurance system for enhancing the scope of healthcare coverage, NHP suggested that a pilot scheme be started to check the social insurance scheme where the

healthcare services are provided by the private sector, and based on outcomes, a policy for insurance be formulated.
- NHP considered the adoption of information technology and recognised the immense potential of telemedicine in the tertiary care sector.
- NHP felt that it had become difficult to implement certain components of the national programmes through the public health machinery and the participation of non-governmental organizations and other civil society organizations have contributed to these programmes, and suggested, that disease control programmes earmark 10 percent of their budgets of identified programme components which should be exclusively implemented through NGOS /CSOs. States would encourage NGOs and other civil society organizations participation for managing public health service outlets.
- NHP considers that the national disease surveillance infrastructure is grossly inadequate and is limited only to the district level which leads to delay in the receipt of the information and is a systemic short coming. NHP envisioned setting up of a fully integrated disease surveillance network with a bottom-up approach, starting from the lowest rung of public health up to the central government by 2005. This would include information from private healthcare institutions as well have real time information to augment the public health system to be prepared to handle the outbreaks of seasonal diseases.
- With regards to health statistics, NHP felt that the absence of a scientific database & a proper national health accounts is a major deficiency. NHP envisioned the setting of a system for baseline estimates for the incidence of common diseases by 2005, and replicating it for non-communicable diseases in the future, and this would lead to evidence-based policy making system. NHP also emphasised the need for setting up of the national health accounts system complying to the 'source- to- users' matrix structure. Also, NHP envisioned the estimation of health costs on regular basis, and these would help in decision making based on the priorities and the financial resources for health sector.
- NHP considered women's health critical to improving the overall health of the population and committed to giving highest priority for programmes related to women's health from the central government. Also, recommended to review the staffing norms to meet the requirements of women's healthcare needs in a more comprehensive manner.

- NHP dwelled on the issue of medical ethics and termed the professional practice scenario as grossly commercial. NHP envisioned that a contemporary code of ethics be implemented by the Medical Council of India, and a vigilant watch on the medical research and the existing guidelines and statutory provisions be reviewed regularly and updated.
- NHP considered the issue of quality standards for foods and drugs and stated the strengthening of the FDA, and the food standards be at par with the best in the world.
- Regulation of paramedics: As there were institutions imparting training without any regulations or monitoring, so, NHP recommended setting up of the statutory professional councils for paramedical disciplines.
- Environmental and occupational health: the NHP felt that environmental conditions pose a significant risk to general health of the population. Also, that work conditions in the country are sub-standard and are a long-term risk of chronic morbidities. NHP envisioned policies and programs of environment to converge with the policies and programmes of healthcare, and there should be regular screening of health conditions of workers, especially for the occupational risks.
- NHP considered the issue of medical tourism for allopathic and ISM and granting the medical tourism services fiscal incentives and also considered giving medical tourism the status of 'deemed exports'.
- NHP looked at the impact of globalization, the post TRIPS era to ensure health security in the country with regards to the cost of medicines and proposed the national patent regime which, while conforming to the TRIPS regimes avails of the opportunities to safeguard the country under its patent laws, and ensure affordable access to the latest medical and other therapeutic developments and set out that the government will use its influence to ensure that the healthcare sector does not faces the adverse impact of the TRIPS regime.
- NHP looked at the inter-sectoral collaboration for health.
- NHP considered population stabilization important for overall development of the people and expressed that the synchronised implementation of the National Population policy 2000 with the National Health Policy 2002 would lead to the improvement of health standards of the population.
- NHP focussed on the need of increased outlays for health and improvement in health infrastructure. Since the issue is paucity of funds, the NHP prioritises the areas of focus

> *like; the diseases that contribute to the major disease burden, rationalising resource allocation with an overarching principle to ensure health equity as an independent goal ,and committing that the centre takes the financial burden of assuring basic health needs of the population, increased participation of private sector ,NGOs , CSOs (Civil Society Organizations) . Also, the improvement in health conditions depended significantly on population stabilization and efforts from other social sectors, empathetic & committed attitude of service providers (both private and public) and improved governance standards* (Gupta R. P., Health Care Reforms in India: Making up for the Lost Decades, 2016, pp. 255-61).

Despite all the above , *"NHP 2002 'does not claim to be a road-map for meeting all the health needs of the populace of the country"* (Gupta R. P., Healthcare Reforms in India: Making up for the lost decades, 2016, p. 260), and this puts a serious question mark on the policy planners and implementors on the overall impact of the NHP-2002 on giving a direction, and addressing the issues facing the healthcare.

Also, the NHP-2002 was silent on the 'comprehensive and universal healthcare' which was the goal of NHP-1983 through its commitment to 'Health for All by 2000' , and the policy was also silent on the village health worker, with nothing substantive on population control, and the primary healthcare (Gupta A. S., 2002).

The policy fell short on its recommendations for women's and children's health (Gupta A. S., 2002).

The NHP-2002 failed to mention about the drug prices and policy and it is not surprising that the country now stands at the crossroads where we are dependent on China for APIs!

If we consider the goals set forth in the National Health Policy (NHP) – 2002, it was stated that Kala-azar will be eliminated by the year 2010; and if we look back at the health policy document in 2017, it was mentioned, 'to achieve and maintain elimination of status of Kala-azar by 2017' (Ministry of Health & Family Welfare, Government of India, 2017, p. 4).

NHP 2002 aimed to bring down the prevalence of blindness to less than 0.5 percent by 2010, and again in National Health Policy -2017, it was mentioned 'to bring down the prevalence of blindness to 0.25 /1000 by 2025, and reduce the disease burden by one third from the current levels (Ministry of Health & Family Welfare, Government of India, 2017, p. 5).

NHP 2002 had set a goal to eliminate Leprosy by 2005, and again in National Health Policy-2017, it was mentioned, 'to achieve and maintain elimination status of Leprosy by 2018' (Ministry of Health & Family Welfare, Government of India, 2017, p. 4)

The issues that were taken up by the earlier health policy (2002) were repeated in the NHP-2017 and the goal posts were moved ahead, because of the failure to achieve the targets as adopted by the earlier National Health Policy-2002. The NHP-2002 had failed to deliver on the above mentioned and perhaps, more!

HLEG Report 2010

In 2010, the Planning Commission of India set up the High-Level Expert Group (HLEG) on Universal Health Coverage (UHC) to work on developing an outline on how to provide easily accessible and affordable healthcare in India. It was assessed that along with financial security, there was a need of adequate healthcare infrastructure, skilled workforce and cost-effective drugs and technologies for achieving the Universal Health Coverage.

HLEG performed a situational analysis of the existing health system and made recommendations to meet the objectives of UHC. It aimed to bridge the gaps and to meet the future health care needs. This group sought advice from Indian and international organizations inclusive of policymakers, health professionals, civil society, private sector, and academicians. Consultations with the members of the Planning Commission also enriched the group's work.

HLEG's recommendations were formed considering the experiences of other countries.

The objectives of HLEG were as follows:

Universal Health Coverage (UHC): To enable quality health care for every citizen of this country, which is equitable; regardless of gender, caste or religion, economic status, and social status. The government serves to guarantee and be an enabler of affordable, accountable, and appropriate health services of good quality.

The terms of reference of HLEG included besides others; creating a detailed roadmap of human resources for health in India, plan the financial norms for ensuring quality, universal and accessible healthcare services across the country, suggest reforms to improve efficiency and accountability of healthcare, identify pathways for engagement of the private and not-for-profit sector in healthcare delivery, develop systems to address the issue of drugs, vaccine and other medical supplies while reducing the cost to the consumer, address the issue of financial provisioning to ensure the universal health coverage and to address the social determinants of health for UHC.
(Planning Commission of India, 2011).

The key recommendations in the HLEG report were as follows:

1. Increase public health expenditures to at least 2.5 percent by the end of the 12th five-year plan, and at least to 3 percent of GDP by 2022.
2. Ensure the availability of essential medicines for free by increasing drug procurement.
3. Healthcare financing through general taxation, along with mandatory deductions for healthcare from salaries of people paying taxes or earning.
4. No sector-specific taxes for financing.
5. No fees while using healthcare services.
6. Introduce mechanisms to ensure equal spending on health across states to reduce hurdles in resource mobilisation.
7. Flexible and differential norms while allocating finances across different states after accounting for the physical, sociocultural, and other differences.
8. At least 70 percent of all healthcare expenditures should go towards primary healthcare, information dissemination, promotion, curative services, risk factor screening and cost-effective treatment.
9. To not utilize the insurance model (companies and agents) to purchase healthcare services on behalf of the government.
10. Central and state governments or attached or quasi-governmental autonomous agencies should be tasked to disburse services under UHC.
11. The UHC system should enable the integration of all government-funded insurance schemes.

12. Every citizen should be offered a National Health Package that includes the basic (essential) health services at all levels of the health care.

13. Private sector services be governed with adequate guidelines and quality checks.

14. Primary healthcare should be the focus of the health care delivery system.

15. District hospitals should be strengthened.

16. Guarantee equitable access to secondary and tertiary care through access to functional beds.

17. Adhere to quality standards across levels and providers.

18. Focus and enable equitable access to healthcare in urban areas.

19. Ensure ample trained healthcare providers and other personnel at all levels to achieve WHO norms for doctors, nurses, and midwives.

20. Make amends to the existing curricula, and introduce continuing education programs to improve the quality of human resources for education and training.

21. Invest in building health workforce.

22. Establish District Health Knowledge Institutes (DHKIs).

23. Increase adequately trained faculty and faculty-sharing across institutions by strengthening State and Regional Institutes of Family Welfare.

24. Train the CHWs.

25. Set up Health Science Universities in every state.

26. Set up the National Council for Human Resources in Health (NCHRH).

27. Transform the Village Health Committees.

28. Organise Health Assemblies.

29. Increase the participation and responsibilities of elected representatives at the local bodies.

30. Civil society and non-governmental organisations should be strengthened.

31. Establishing a grievance redressal mechanism at the block level.

32. Regulating the price of essential drugs.

33. Essential Drugs List should be amended and revised.

34. Enhance the capacity of local manufacturing as per domestic needs.

35. Ensure the rational use of drugs.

36. State and National drug supply logistics corporations should be established.

37. The Indian patents law and the TRIPS Agreement should be upheld to protect the country's needs with regards to essential drugs, etc.

38. The drug regulatory system should be strengthened.

39. Establish a Public Health Service Cadre and at the state level, a specialized state level Health Systems Management Cadres.

40. Improve recruitment, better performance, motivation to continue by rationalizing pay and incentives; and introduce career tracking by a competency-based assessment method.

41. Ensure inter-operability across healthcare stakeholders by developing a national health information technology network.

42. To establish a strong relationship between management and regulatory systems to ensure accountability to care seekers.

43. For streamlining the fund flow, establish financing and budgeting systems.

44. Recommended the setting up of various regulatory agencies.

45. Increase the investments across health sciences research and innovation to guide policy, programmes and recommend practical solutions (High Level Expert Group Report on Universal Health Coverage for India, 2011).

Various Committees on Health

Since 1943 till 2011, India had 23 commissions, committees, and reports on health for which the reports are available, and there are additional committees, for which the reports are not available (Gupta R. P., Health Care Reforms in India: Making up for the Lost Decades, 2016, pp. 164-5). List of committees for which the report is available are listed below.

1. Health Survey and Development Committee – Bhore Committee 1946.
2. Report of the National Planning Committee – Subcommittee on National Health – Sokhey Committee 1948.
3. Dave Committee 1955.
4. K.N. Udupa Committee on Ayurveda Research Evaluation 1959.
5. Health Survey and Planning Committee (Lakshmanaswami Mudaliar Committee), Government of India, 1961.
6. Report of the Special Committee on the Preparation of Entry of the National Malaria Education Programme into the Maintenance of Phase- Chadha Committee, DGHS, Ministry of Health, New Delhi 1963.
7. Mukherjee Committee Report on Basic Health Services, Government of India, 1966.
8. Committee Appointed to Review Staffing Pattern and Financial Provision under Family Planning Programme, Government of India, 1966.

9. Report of the Committee on Integration of Health Services (Jungalwala Committee) 1966.
10. Report of the Committee on Multipurpose Workers under Health and Family Welfare Programme (Kartar Singh Committee), Government of India, 1973.
11. Report of the Group on Medical Education and Support Manpower, Health Services and Medical Education – A Programme for Immediate Action, Government of India, 1973.
12. Report of the Consultative Committee of Experts to Determine Alternative Strategies under National Malaria Eradication Programme (NMEP), 1974.
13. Report of the Committee on Drugs and Pharmaceuticals Industry (Hathi Committee), Government of India, 1980.
14. Report of the working Group on Population Policy, Planning Commission, Government of India, 1981.
15. Report of the Working Group on 'Health for All' by the year 2020 AD, MoHFW, Government of India, 1981.
16. Report of the Medical Education Review Committee (Mehta Committee), Government of India, 1983.
17. Report of the Expert Committee on Health Manpower Planning, Production and Management (Bajaj Committee), Government of India, 1987.
18. Report of the High-Power Committee on Nursing and Nursing Profession, Government of India, 1989.
19. Report of the Expert Committee on Public Health System (Bajaj Committee), Government of India, 1996.
20. Report of the Task Force on Conservation and Sustainable Use of Medicinal Plants, 2000.
21. Report of the Committee on Drugs Regulatory Issues (Mashelkar Committee), 2003.
22. Report of the National Commission on Macroeconomics and Health, 2005.
23. High Level Expert Group on Universal Health Coverage (HLEG), 2011.

Health and Human Development Report 2020

The first Human Development Report was released over three decades ago and introduced the Human Development Index (HDI), this is a measure of human progress to assess people's freedom to live the life they decide to live. It also assesses the population's average longevity, education, and income.

India falls in the medium human development category with the HDI value for 2019 at 0.645 and is ranked at 131 out of 189. In the past two decades (till 2019), the life expectancy at birth in India has increased by 11.8 years, access to education increased by 3.5 mean years and 4.5 years increase in expected years of schooling was observed.

Another measure of health in the HDR is the GDI (Gender Development Index) and it is the relationship between gender-based inequalities in achieving three key parameters of human development: health, education, and the command over economic resources. In 2019, India was placed in Group 5 with female HDI value of 0.573 and 0.699 for males.

In 2010, reproductive health, empowerment, and economic activity were introduced as the measures of gender-based inequalities (GII). Maternal mortality rate and the adolescent birth rates are the measures of reproductive health India in 2019 was ranked 123 out of 162 with a GII value of 0.488. In India, for every 100,000 live births, pregnancy related complications for 133.0 deaths.

In 2010, the Multidimensional Poverty Index (MPI) with three dimensions, that is, health, education and standard of living was introduced by HDR. Household surveys are the base of MPI. All the dimensions are measured to create deprivation scores that are compared between individuals in the survey. If the value is higher than 33.3 percent, the whole household is classified as multidimensionally poor.

In India, as of 2015-16, according to the MPI, about 27.9 percent of the population (377,492 thousand people) were multidimensionally poor and suffer from deprivations in health, education, and standard of living (Human Development Reports, 2020).

National Health Policy 2017

The burden of healthcare is increasing and becoming complicated with time, and this calls for a bottom-up and inclusive process in defining the health policies. The National Health Policy released in 2017 has attempted to address the complexities of the emerging healthcare scenario.

India, now the world's second-most populous country, is home to around 18 percent of the global population. To give a sense of the complexity of India's healthcare with regards to the population, India's population is equal to the combined population of six nations, namely USA, Indonesia, Brazil, Pakistan, Bangladesh, and Japan (Kalita A. et al., 2015). Large human resource bases, on the other hand, come with a host of problems. Malnutrition, cleanliness, vaccination, sanitation, and infectious diseases are major health problems in India's underdeveloped regions; on the other side, lifestyle diseases and environmental health and other non-communicable diseases, are causing worry in the developed regions. Cardiovascular illnesses, cancer, Tuberculosis (TB), malaria, diabetes, dengue fever, respiratory infections, chikungunya, water, and vector-borne diseases remain important issues in the latter group. Emerging infectious illnesses including; severe acute respiratory syndrome (SARS), Ebola, swine flu (H1N1) influenza and virus-related disorders are an added concern. Central Bureau of Health Intelligence (CBHI) reports that India is grappling with the 'triple burden of diseases,' which is besides the unfinished agenda for infectious diseases as well as the new infectious disease threats (Central Bureau of health Intelligence. National Health Profile 2016). Currently, India is the world's fourth-largest economy, and is expanding rapidly. India has made considerable progress in various health indicators, from the life expectancy to infant and maternal mortality rates, as well as the overall death rate (Planning Commission. Report of the steering committee on health for the 12th five-year plan. Health division, Government of India. [Internet] 2012).

1. The birth rate is also declining. Currently there are large number of physicians, health clinics, and nursing homes to serve the country's rural areas, though a lot more are needed, given that India falls short on doctors to population ratio. The effectiveness of these programmes may be ascribed to the increased penetration of healthcare services, enhanced vaccination, and increased literacy, as well as other government and private sector initiatives. The insurance industry has made a significant contribution to

improvement of health. There has been an increase in the number of private players since health insurance was liberalised, but 74 percent of the insurance is still provided through different government-sponsored programmes and schemes. It was 1.12 percent of GDP in 2009–10, but that number was just one-tenth of a percent lower in 2010–11. About one percent of the GDP was spent on public health in 2013–14 (Bajpai, 2018).

2. It's noted in the National Health Policy (NHP)-2017 background paper that the private healthcare businesses include 15 percent insurance and equipment, 25 percent medicines, and 10 percent diagnostics, with a total value of 40 billion dollars, with a projected increase to 220 billion dollars by 2020. The government, on the other hand, has made significant investments in the healthcare industry by lowering direct taxes, increasing depreciation on medical equipment, and providing rural hospitals with five years of income tax exemptions as well as exemptions from customs duties on life-saving equipment (Government of India. Situation analysis: backdrop to the national health policy 2017, World Health Organization. World health statistics. [Internet] 2010).

3. In comparison to other densely populated developing nations and industrialised countries, India spends a small fraction of its GDP on healthcare. In 2019, India spent 3.5 percent of its GDP on health care sector (Duggal R., 2001). The investment on public sector was lowest when compared to other countries (44.70 percent). In the private sector, India spent the highest (73.80 percent), whereas worldwide average was 40.40 percent. In India, the healthcare sector is expanding due to population growth, the projected rise in geriatric people and lifestyle-related illnesses, increasing adoption of digital health, as well as increased literacy and disposable money that makes health care more accessible to the public.

After a long gap of fourteen years, in 2017, the union cabinet approved the National Health Policy, which has transformed the context of healthcare in multiple ways. The increasing incidence of communicable and non-communicable diseases; the exponential growth of the private sector; higher health expenditure along with the economic growth that enabled improved fiscal strength has its influence on the formulation of the National Health Policy in 2017. The NHP-2017 guaranteed quality health care to everyone. There was a transition from sickness to wellness in people in the overall approach of the NHP-2017.

Focus areas of NHP-2017

The key objective of the National Health Policy, 2017, is to provide information with clarity on the Government's role in shaping the country's health systems including health investments, healthcare services organization, disease prevention and promoting good health through cross sectoral approach, using technology, human resources development, building knowledge base, and good financial protection strategies. NHP-2017 was formulated considering the developments since the previous health policy released in 2002. The developments have been captured in the 'Situation Analysis' which has been put as a separate document besides the National Health Policy- 2017.

The objective of NHP-2017 was to strive towards improving the health status via coordinated policy approach across all sectors and increase access to preventive, promotive, curative, palliative, and rehabilitative management with focus on quality.

The key policy principles were as follows:

I. Professionalism, Integrity and Ethics: The policy has assured the highest professional standards, integrity, and ethics across the health care delivery, that will be evaluated by a credible, transparent, and responsible regulatory system.
II. Equity: The policy aims at reducing inequity by catering to even the poorest. No distinction based on gender, poverty, caste, disability, other forms of social exclusion and geographical barriers.
III. Affordability: With increasing cost, affordability will be addressed.
IV. Universality: No distinctions for availing healthcare services.
V. Patient-centred and Quality of Care: All services will be gender sensitive, safe, effective, and will be provided with confidentiality and dignity.
VI. Accountability: accountability of financial transactions and performance, transparency in decision making, and eliminating corruption.
VII. Inclusive Partnerships: A multistakeholder approach towards addressing all health care issues by involving partnership and participation even among non-health ministries and communities.
VIII. Pluralism: Patients have the right to choose AYUSH care.

IX. Decentralization: After practical considerations and based on institutional capacity, decentralisation of decision making will be achieved. Policy aims to promote the role of community in healthcare planning.

X. Dynamism and Adaptiveness: Health policy aims for constant improvement based on the emerging evidence (National Health Policy, 2017).

The Make in India concept regulated medicine and equipment manufacture. Special focus was on traditional medicine-Ayurveda, Yoga, Unani, Siddha and Homeopathy (AYUSH), particularly yoga. Besides the NHPs, numerous additional policies that are closely connected to enhancing the health of individuals have been introduced from time to time (Table 3). Given that the National Health Policy 2017 is less than five years into implementation, it may be too early to take a call on the effectiveness of the policy, but given the structured launch of the PM-JAY with the initiation of the National Health Authority and the Ayushman Bharat Digital Mission, the direction and focus of the new health policy is assuring from its institutionalised approach for implementation of key recommendations.

Table 3: National health policies/other related policies for promotion of health

Year	Name of Policy
1983	National Health Policy
1992	National AIDS Control and Prevention Policy
1993	National Nutrition Policy
1999	National Policy on Older Persons
2000	National Population Policy
2001	National Policy for Empowerment of Women
2002	National Blood Policy
2002	National Policy on Indian System of Medicine and Homeopathy
2002	National Health Policy
2003	National Policy for Access to Plasma-derived Medicinal Products from Human Plasma for Clinical/Therapeutic use
2003	National charter for children
2005	National Rural Health Mission
2006	National Environment Policy
2009	Right of children to Free and Compulsory Education Bill—2009 (education to children aged between 6 and 14 years)
2012	National Pharmaceutical Pricing Policy
2012	National Water Policy
2013	National Policy for Children
2015	National Youth Policy
2017	National Health Policy
2020	National Education Policy

Table 4 and 5 depicts other national policies which address the issue of various diseases

Table 4: National Health Programmes

Year	Name of Programme
1955	National Leprosy Eradication Programme (NLEP)
1955	National Filaria Control Programme (NFCP)
1962	National TB Control Programme (NTC)
1978	Immunization Programme (Renamed as UIP in 1985)
1983	National Guinea Worm Eradication Programme (NGEP)
	National Vector Borne Disease Control Programme (NVBDCP)
1990	National AIDS Control Programme (NACP)
1992	Revised National TB Control Programme (RNTCP)
1993	Yaws Control Programme
1996	Integrated Disease Surveillance Projects (IDSP)
2000	Voluntary Blood Donation Programme (VBDP)

Table 5: National Health Programmes for NCDs

Year	Name of Programme
1950s	National STD Control Programme
1962	National Goitre Control Programme (NGCP)
1975	National Cancer Control Programme (NCCP)/National Programme for Prevention and Control of Cancer (NPPCC)
1976	National Programme for Control of Blindness (NPCB)
1982	National Cancer Registry Programme (NCRP)
1982	National Mental Health Programme (NMHP)
1988	Drug De addiction Programme (DDAP), Revised in 1993
1992	National Goitre Control Programme (NGCP) was renamed National Iodine Deficiency Disorder Control Programme (NIDDCP)
1992	National AIDS Control Programme (NACP)
1995	Pulse Polio Immunisation programme
1996	District Mental Health Programme
1998	National Programme for Control and Treatment of Occupational Diseases (NPCTOD)
2006	National Programme for Prevention and Control of Deafness (NPPCD)
2007	National Tobacco Control Programme (NTCP)
2008	National Programme for Prevention and Control of Fluorosis (NPPCF)
2010	National Programme on Prevention and Control of Diabetes, CVD and Stroke
2010	National Programme for Health Care in Elderly (NPHCE)
2014	National Oral Health Programme

Apart from this, in 2006, Pradhan Mantri Swasthya Suraksha Yojana (PMSSY), Janani Shishu Suraksha Karyakram, and Janani Suraksha Yojana were established by Ministry of Health and Family Welfare for health insurance. Various programmes were also initiated by the Ministry for Social Justice and Empowerment, and the Ministry of Women and Child Development such as, the Integrated Child Development Services (ICDS), the Midday Meal (MDM) Programme, and the Reproductive and Child Health (RCH) Programme. The National Drinking Water Mission (RGNDWM) was launched by the Ministry of Drinking Water and Sanitation to provide clean water.

National Rural Health Mission

The National Rural Health Mission (NRHM) was launched on 12th April 2005, to cater to the needs of vulnerable groups and rural population by increasing accessibility, affordability, and quality.

The focus of NRHM was the Empowered Action Group (EAG) States, which includes the North-Eastern States, Jammu and Kashmir and Himachal Pradesh. The mission addressed all areas of health and decentralized health delivery system. It focused on all aspects impacting health. NRHM recognised the strong relationship between adolescent health, family planning, maternal health, and child survival outcomes (National Rural Health Mission (NRHM), 2021).

National Rural Health Mission was absorbed into newly initiated National Health Mission (NHM) and is considered a sub-mission of National Health Mission (NHM) alongside National Urban Health Mission (NUHM). ASHA, which is one of NHMs most successful aspect, helped to bring health awareness to most of the rural population while also assisting in making the mission more decentralised. It also aided in the participation of the rural masses in designing of the health system based on their own health settings. The states have set the goal of achieving 'Health for All' by subsuming National Rural Health Mission into the National Health Mission.

There has been a steady decline on the key metrics according to the Census of India's Sample Registration System (SRS) report, the Maternal Mortality Ratio (MMR) had declined from 130 per 100,000 live births in SRS 2014-16 to 122 in SRS 2015-17 and 113 in SRS 2016-18

(Ministry of Health and Family Welfare, Government of India, 2021). With this success in lowering the MMR, India has made definite progress and is on the way to achieving the SDG of 70 lakh live births by 2030.

India had reduced its total fertility rate to 2.0 from 2.2 in 2015-16 (Ministry of Health & Family Welfare, Government of India, 2022), which is lower than the NRR of 2.1, while the global average set by WHO is 2.1. In terms of reduction rate, the EAG states are catching up with other states, but the disparity remains significant. As per the annual report of the Ministry of Health and Family Welfare for 2013-14 (National Health Mission, 2018), institutional deliveries increased to more than 1 crore from around 7.3 lakhs in 2005, and by 2014, around 8.5 crore women benefited from this. The National Family Health Survey states, 89 percent of rural women delivered under the care of a skilled personnel (NFHS-4 Report, 2015-16).

According to the latest round of NFHS-5 (2019-21), the institutional births have increased to 88.6 (Ministry of Health & Family Welfare, Government of India, 2022), and it was 78.9 in the earlier round of NFHS (NFHS-4). Countering communicable and noncommunicable diseases is the most significant burden on the community in the absence of proper sanitation, hygiene, and nutritional intake. Even though the National Rural Health Mission has made significant contributions to addressing this issue, India is still struggling to achieve the desired results due to low sanitation levels, unhygienic practices, and poor nutrition. The mission determinants such as hygiene, drinking water, and sanitation have partially achieved the goals, but there are targets remaining to be met for 100 percent achievement. Nutrition influences children's health indicators and impacts the future burden of NCDs. Basic vaccinations increased at a higher rate in rural India when compared to urban India. The increase across rural India ranges from 39 percent to 61 percent, while in urban scenario it ranges from 58 percent to 64 percent (National Rural Health Mission.2020).

To achieve global health standards, the objectives of the National Rural Health Mission fall short on functionality, training and the utilisation of ASHA workers, as well as proper implementation of all other components of the mission, and fails to deliver proper health interventions to the rural population, and assist in the long-term development. Furthermore, the aim of Universal

Health Coverage may be achieved through the recent scheme "Ayushman Bharat", which has emerged as part of the process of reforming the health care system. If implemented well, the program can reduce the out-of-pocket expenditure and thus increase India's growth and development (National Rural Health Mission, 2020).

National Urban Health Mission (NUHM)

The National health policy not only recognizes but also lays high emphasis on the primary health care needs of the population living in the urban areas, and gives special emphasis on poor living in slums, and other vulnerable communities. To address the growing urban health challenges, the policy advocated expanding the NUHM to include the entire urban population. Policy also prioritized the utilization of AYUSH professionals in managing the healthcare needs of urban areas. Given the prominent existence of the private sector in urban areas, policy suggested exploring the possibility of developing viable models of private public partnership for urban health care delivery. Convergence of the larger determinants of health was also the focus of urban health mission. The NUHM also addresses the healthcare needs of people living in semiurban areas. Furthermore, non-communicable diseases (NCDs), including diabetes and hypertension, prevalent in urban areas, were addressed by NUHM. Improved secondary prevention was also a key component of the NUHM. Improved health seeking behaviour, capacity building of community-based organisations and creating a referral mechanism, were also key recommendations of the policy (National Health Policy 2017).

Issues and Challenges of NUHM

1. NUHM has been a hope for country's urban poor. However, no systematic exercise was conducted prior to the mission's implementation to assess the gaps in healthcare delivery for the urban areas. Even though the mission cites studies to assess the health problems of the urban poor, but the studies were not conducted in a systematic manner with proper scientific sampling.

2. In rural areas, there is a well-defined system across the country, whereas the urban areas have very sophisticated administrative structures. Urban administrative structures are broadly classified as; town panchayats, municipalities, municipal corporations, and the urban local bodies, and so on. As a result, service planning and implementation must be distinct. This complicates the operational design and delivery of services to urban areas.

3. The mission's framework makes no mention of health insurance services. People in cities have the highest OOPE.

4. The mission is more skewed towards female participation. The common health and social problems necessitate the presence of male health workers/activists in the programme.

5. Even though the mission framework includes all vulnerable groups in urban areas such as rag pickers, rickshaw pullers, etc, The missions fails to address the logistics associated with healthcare delivery. An institutional framework is missing!

6. While there is a strong emphasis on public-private partnerships, the issues related to addressing the quality gaps remains unaddressed.

7. In India, the poverty line is viewed as a "magic rope", with political and administrative bodies pulling or pushing the rope in either direction to inflate or deflate the burden of poverty.

8. Non-communicable diseases, substance abuse, mental illnesses, and lifestyle interventions necessitate specific strategies that address these issues adequately.

9. The mission makes no provision for sub-centres. All cases are be referred to UPHCs located far away from these areas.

10. There are difficulties in recruiting doctors in rural areas, as well as the urban slums, as qualified individuals residing in urban areas prefer other options than the government services unless we revisit the norms in government service (Kulkarni P., 2014).

National Health Mission (NHM)

The National Health Mission (NHM) was launched by the Government of India in 2013. This mission subsumed NRHM and NUHM.

The mission has played a key role in the decline of MMR, IMR, U5MR, and TFR. This has also positively impacted the various disease programmes.

The various new initiatives under the National Health Mission 2019-2020 have been added for social awareness and action to reduce deaths because of childhood pneumonia, free services for maternal and neonatal health under a single scheme, training of nurse practitioners in midwifery for RMNCH services, and to promote health through school amongst students.

Implementation strategy and targets

Implementation strategy:

The implementation strategy of Ministry of Health and Family Welfare under NHM is to provide financial and technical support to States / Union Territories (UTs) enabling them to provide accessible, affordable, accountable, and effective healthcare up to District Hospitals (DHs), especially to the poor and vulnerable sections of the population. It has also aimed to bridge the gap in rural healthcare services through improved health infrastructure, augmentation of human resource and improved service delivery in rural areas and has envisaged decentralization of programme to district level to facilitate need-based interventions, improve intra and inter-sectoral convergence and effective utilization of resources.

Targets for NHM:

- Aims to reduce the MMR, IMR to 1/1000, 25/1000 live births.
- To reduce TFR to 2.1.
- Reduce the prevalence and incidence of Leprosy, and malaria.
- Prevent the reduce the mortality and morbidity due to NCDs.
- To reduce the OOPE.
- To end tuberculosis by 2025.

Expenditure: *Rs 27,989.00 Cr (Central Share.* The scheme is aimed for the entire population through the public health facilities. (Ministry of Health & Family Welfare, Government of India, 2021).

Sustainable Development Goals – SDGs

Post the Millennium Development Goals (MDGs), which had a mixed bag of success, the UN has come up with the idea and adopted the Sustainable Development Goals (SDGs).

"The Sustainable Development Goals (SDGs) are also referred as the Global Goals. These goals were adopted by the United Nations in 2015 as a global call to action to end poverty, protect the planet, and ensure that by 2030 all people enjoy peace and prosperity and based on the overarching theme of sustainability.

There are a total of seventeen SDGs, and they are integrated goals. The SDGs recognize the interdependence of the goals and aim for a development based on social, economic and environmental sustainability. SDG-3 is about Good Health and Well-Being, SDG-6 is about clean water and sanitation (UNDP, 2021).

India is a signatory to the SDGs and has mentioned about the crucial importance of the SDGs and mentions about the time bound and quantitative goals which are aligned to the global strategic direction in the very beginning of the Health Policy (Ministry of Health & Family Welfare, Government of India, 2017, p. 1).

Economic Survey – 2020-21

Every year, just before the budget, an annual document, a survey is presented by the Ministry of Finance. The Chief Economic Advisor of India guides the writing of this document. In 1950-51, the first Economic Survey of India was presented. The document studies the Indian economy and the contributing factors in the past financial year and presents it before the budget.

This document guides health policy decisions for the current financial year as health and financial development are inter-related (Finlay, 2007).

The government launched the Pradhan Mantri Jan Arogya Yojana (PM-JAY) in 2018, which aims to provide healthcare services to population living below poverty line (BPL). This scheme has contributed significantly on the healthcare outcomes of the states that have implemented the scheme. The following causal effects of PM-JAY on health outcomes were discovered:

Improved health-care coverage: the impact of the scheme can be gauged from the fact that across all states, the proportion of households with health insurance increased by 54 percent in states that have implemented PMJAY, whereas, it has decreased by 10 percent in states that did not.

Infant Mortality Rate (IMR): In case of IMR, the impact is clearly visible. This has decreased by 12 percent in states that did not implement PM-JAY and by 20 percent in states that implemented the scheme. Deaths among children under the age of five are on the decline. The comparison shows that states that implemented PM-JAY saw significant improvements in several health outcomes compared to those that did not.

Inequality and Growth: The National Health Mission (NHM) was critical in reducing inequity by increasing access of the poorest to prenatal/postnatal care and institutional deliveries.

Key Healthcare Policy Suggestions:

(a) Emphasis on NHM in conjunction with Ayushman Bharat should keep going.

(b) Increase in government healthcare spending from 1 percent to 2.5-3.0 percent of GDP, which will reduce out-of-pocket spending from 65 percent to 35 percent of total healthcare spending.

(c) A healthcare regulatory body must be considered.

(d) Mitigation of information asymmetry to aid in the reduction of insurance premiums and the provision of better products.

(e) Broaden insurance coverage.

(f) Telemedicine must be implemented (Highlights of Economic Survey 2020- 2021. 2021).

Challenges in Health Policy Making Process in India

In a lower-middle-income country like India, balancing between priorities and resource allocation while formulating health policy is plagued by difficult choices. Other than the barriers in the health system, many other factors come into the picture while designing a health policy for a diverse and pluralistic country like India. The current policy making scenario demonstrates how the health policy in India is not evidence based but eminence based (influenced by powerful activist groups and people close to power centres) and for electoral gains. The priority for any issue is mostly based on what is on the highest priority of the political agenda rather than what is the ground reality and a public concern. For instance, deaths by snake bites and self-harm by consuming pesticides are not addressed because these conditions mostly affect the poor, and marginalised population with a feeble political voice and therefore genuine healthcare needs are neglected.

Policies that do not consider good quality evidence to back the decisions made in the policy result in causing problems in the growth and development of a country. One prominent example of this faulty decision making was the public interest litigation accusing those vaccines with no utility and which compromised safety and efficacy. It also pointed out that unnecessary vaccinations had replaced six basic vaccines that were very important.

Another example of change in health care decisions not based on evidence was banning the use of pioglitazone based on a letter from a prominent diabetologist and not on any meta-analysis or systematic review. Incidents like these lead to controversies and confrontations that can result in selective citation of scientific evidence to fulfil needs of the participants involved in policy making.

Examples demonstrating the benefits of evidence-based health policy decisions

There are great examples of evidence-based decisions in the health policy that improved health care outcomes in India. After the Tsunami disaster in 2004, there was a debate on the type of intervention that should be administered to combat post-traumatic stress disorder. The benefits of mass sensitization approach by passing information as a speech to the entire village versus identifying high risk individuals were compared. Evidence based on a systematic review showed that identifying high risk individuals and treating them was a better approach when compared to mass briefing. This also led to the development of the Evidence Aid arm.

Designing and modifying health care programmes to address problems not only involves factors such as financial limitations, time constraints, administrative and technical capability, but also factors such as political agenda and the vested interests.

Relevance of evidence-based policy making to the Indian context

There is a demographic shift in the Indian population towards an urban, educated, and well-informed society that understands and questions the changes in the health policy. With the implementation of the Right to Information Act, and Lokpal Bill, need was felt for the government to monitor the ground level impact of the health policies in a transparent, and systematic process. A well-developed policy assessment mechanism is required to address the needs and expectations of citizens while also ensuring the effective utilization of the resources and the quality of services (Bhaumik S., 2014).

Challenges

A range of contrasting landscapes is depicted in the Indian health situation. At one end of the scale, the glittery buildings provide the metropolitan Indian people with high-end healthcare. At the other side, the dilapidated buildings in the far regions of the country are urgently seeking refurbishment to be identified as health facilities and wait to be turned in sanctuaries of health and wellbeing. This spectrum will probably continue to expand in the future, with the high speed of change now underway.

Four "A" challenges include -

Awareness or the lack of it: Awareness studies are multiple and varied, but awareness gaps seem to spread over our country's life span. In two studies, barely a third of pregnant women had enough understanding on breastfeeding (Taraphdar et al., 2016, Pandey et al., 2015).

Research in urban Haryana revealed that just 11.3 percent of teenagers surveyed recognised the main problems of reproductive health accurately (Mittal, K. and Goel, M.K., 2010) A review of geriatric morbidity study revealed that only 20.3 percent of respondents were aware of underlying causes behind the commonly occurring diseases and their prevention (Tamanna, M.Z., et al. 20212). This paucity of awareness can be attributed to poor education, inadequate functional literacy, low emphasis on health system education, and low population health priority, among others. But the evidence shows that the attempts to increase awareness are typically successful. For example, in a study from Bihar and Jharkhand, awareness and views about abortion improved following an intervention on behavioural changes (Banerjee, S.K, et al. 2013). An evaluation of the efficacy of teenage reproductive health treatments has demonstrated a substantial improvement in the awareness of women wellness, environmental health, nutritional awareness, and reproductive and child health (RCH), after intervention (Kotwal N et al. 2014).

Access or the lack of it: The dictionary definition (Oxford) of access to healthcare is, "the right or opportunity of (healthcare) usage or benefit" (Oxford Dictionary Online). Once again, the issue "What is the degree of access to decent healthcare?" is highly important if we move beyond the moderately well-connected metropolitan people into the urban poor and their rural equivalents. A 2002 study talks about access as a complicated topic, and talks about accessibility issues, the supply and use of healthcare services as variables. The use of these services even where available services might be limited by barriers to access in economic, organisational, social, and cultural realms (Gulliford, M. et al., 2002).

One of the key dimensions of access is the ability to reach a healthcare facility within five kilometre of the workplace or the residence (Munjanja, S.P et al. 2012). In 2012, a survey conducted in India revealed that just 37 percent of the rural population had access to IPD facilities in a radius of five km, while 68 percent had access to ambulatory services (Understanding Healthcare Access in India. 2012). The farther people live from town, bigger are the risks of sickness, malnutrition, frailty, and premature mortality, as postulated by Krishna and Ananthapur in their 2012 study (Krishna A. and Ananthpur K., 2013). Which grade of treatment does a health institution give even if it is physically accessible? Does this care always exist? A study from six states across the country in 2012 revealed that most of the primary health centres (PHC) lack even the basic infrastructure like; beds, toilets, drinking water installations, clean laboratories, and electricity, this is despite the National Health Mission's efforts to improve infrastructure in the Indian Government (Understanding Healthcare Access in India. 2012).

The human resource crisis in healthcare: Any debate on health care should probably include the most critical element of the 'workforce' or 'competent human resources'. Do we have enough staff, are they properly trained, are they fairly employed and are their moral values relatively high in the provision of service? This workforce is not evenly distributed, most of them working in regions where their family resides, and infrastructure and amenities are better. The economically backward regions of the North and Central India often have lesser health workers than in the southern regions (Rao, M. et al., 2011). While most of the national health spending is through the private sector, most of the country's rural and peri-urban areas still have a state-owned health sector to choose from.

When a person must undertake an arduous journey to reach the point of delivery, the lack of a qualified individual is a major deterrent to people's health care-seeking behaviour. As per the data from the Ayushman Bharat- Health and Wellness Centres, India has 76,663 Health and Wellness Centres (HWCs), Urban Primary Health Centres (UPHCs) stood at 3998 and total number of Primary Health Centres (PHCs) stood at 21081 and the total number of Sub-Health Centres (SHCs) stood at 51,584 (Ministry of Health & Family Welfare, Government of India, 2019). Since the private health sector plays a dominant role in the provision of health care services, a number of initiatives have been conceptualized to use private expertise to provide public health services.

Affordability: The private sector is well recognized as the main player in Indian healthcare. Nearly 75 percent of health spending comes from household bags and the catastrophic health care spending are an important reason of pushing people below the poverty line (Rural health statistics 2019-2020. 2020). According to the WHO (World Health Organization , 2005), a health expenditure is defined as catastrophic, when it is greater than or equal to 40 percent of a household's non-subsistence income, i.e., income available after basic needs have been met.

Furthermore, there is a problem of private sector's lack of regulations and the resulting variance in service quality and pricing. The public sector provides medical services for free but is considered or rather perceived as of poor quality and not of an acceptable standard by the care seekers, and is not usually the first choice unless the private sector services are not available. Local and national initiatives are the solutions to address the issue of affordability of healthcare. Government health spending must be expanded as a matter of urgency from current low levels of 2 percent to between 5-6 percent of the gross national product (Balarajan et al., 2011).

This translates into the much-needed improvement of infrastructure in rural and disadvantaged regions and ideally, better health services, and staff availability. The national health insurance programme should be developed carefully to ensure that the smallest target group members are registered and understand exactly what the plan means to them. Locally, the healthcare industry, from the lowest to the highest level, must be aware of the costs. It should prevent wasteful expenses, alternatives that need significant expenditure, and excessive usage of tests and processes. The average medical student is not exposed to problems of healthcare costs. It is expected that exposing young brains to health economics may perhaps lead to realising that the situation is enormous and there is a necessity to deal with it in the best way possible.

<u>Accountability or the lack of it:</u> The methods and processes by which a party defends and takes responsibility for its conduct have been identified as 'responsible' (Reddy, K.S, 2011).

The policy-making process (PMP) relates to how policies are initiated, formulated, or specified, organised, communicated, executed, and assessed. However, policy change needs a practical adjustment in the rules for new approaches to developing programs with more stringent measurements or modifying criteria. These changes entail a complex process, as policymakers must consider a variety of factors for their decision-making, including evidence of the impact on health, priorities of the stakeholders, feasibility, political and societal factors and their impact on the process, and advocacy group's efforts. Among these, the usage of evidence-based research tools to back the policy decisions is critical in this complicated process of policy formulation.

Methodology

This section aims to explain the materials and methods to study the Health Policy Process in India. It includes the research design used to undertake the survey, inclusion, and exclusion criteria to select the respondents, method to calculate sample size, geographies covered, how the data is collected, and type of questions asked and tools for analysing the responses.

Research Design

The design of the research study is cross-sectional. The survey was conducted which used semi-structured questionnaire. The participants are studied for their awareness and opinions across various domains of Health Policy making process in India. Because of COVID-19, participants are assessed through various time stages (multistage) based on participant's year of experiences as it was impossible to conduct the survey in a single time- frame due to restrictions in movement (lockdown) imposed by Government of India across the country.

Study Population

The study targeted healthcare professionals, lawmakers and various other groups which are the stakeholders in Health Policy making process and participants were selected from the professions related directly or indirectly to health sector (including lawmakers) in India. Study population included the following:

- Member of Indian parliament
- Senior bureaucrats
- Doctors (MBBS, BDS and AYUSH)
- MBBS and AYUSH students
- Other health care professionals (Pharmacists, Nurses, Optometrist, ASHAs, Anganwadi workers, Female Health Workers, Medical Representatives, OT assistants and Laboratory Technicians)
- Representatives from the civil society
- Health care policymakers
- Journalists covering healthcare
- Professional associations (The Indian Medical Association, Indian Public Health Association of India, Telemedicine Society of India, HIMSS etc.)

Exclusion and Inclusion Criteria

All participants were related directly or indirectly to healthcare. Age is not considered for the present study. Individuals with wide range of experience (zero to more than 25 years of experience) were included and distributed across private, public, and non-government organizations at National, State, District and sub-district level.

Those who have no professional affiliation to health were excluded.

Geographies Covered

The participants were recruited from 15 states and 2 Union Territories viz. Bihar, Chandigarh, Delhi, Haryana, Jharkhand, Karnataka, Kerala, Madhya Pradesh, Maharashtra, Nagaland, Odisha, Punjab, Rajasthan, Tripura, Uttar Pradesh, Uttarakhand, and Gujarat. Selection of above states was based on NITI Aayog's State Health Index report titled 'Healthy States, Progressive India' (NITI Aayog, 2019, p. 15). States were further selected from the list based on the convenience of the researcher (Due to COVID restrictions). States represents all North-East-West-South geographies of India.

NITI Aayog's State Health Index classifies 21 Indian states as large states, 8 as small states and 7 as Union Territories.

Categories	Number of States and UTs	States and UTs
Larger States	21	Andhra Pradesh, Assam, Bihar, Chhattisgarh, Gujarat, Haryana, Himachal Pradesh, Jammu and Kashmir, Jharkhand, Karnataka, Kerala, Madhya Pradesh, Maharashtra, Odisha, Punjab, Rajasthan, Tamil Nadu, Telangana, Uttar Pradesh, Uttarakhand, West Bengal
Smaller States	8	Arunachal Pradesh, Goa, Manipur, Meghalaya, Mizoram, Nagaland, Sikkim, Tripura
Union Territories	7	Andaman and Nicobar Islands, Chandigarh, Dadra and Nagar Haveli, Daman and Diu, Delhi, Lakshadweep, Puducherry

Sampling Method

Participants were selected based on purposive sampling at national, state, and district level and across private, public, and non-government organizations. At first, participants having experience of fewer than 5 years were surveyed, followed by people with experience of around 5-10 years, more than 10 and less than 15 years, between 15-20 years and more than 20 years representing all levels in the healthcare delivery systems across states. These included clinicians and non-clinicians, influencers, and stakeholders.

Study Sample Size

The following formula was used for the arriving at the sample size;

$$n = \frac{p(100-p)Z^2}{E^2}$$

Where;

n is the sample size required

p is the percentage occurrence of a state or condition (proportion or prevalence)

E is the percentage maximum error required

Z is the value corresponding to the level of confidence required.

Going with the assumption, that at least 50 percent of the respondents were aware of the health policy process, at 99 percent confidence level and 10 percent of maximum error, the sample size was taken as,

$$n = \frac{50 \times (100-50) \times 2.58^2}{10^2}$$

$$n = 166.41 \approx 166$$

Hence, the minimum sample size required was 166. With the increase in the sample size, the accuracy of the result also increases. Hence the study recruited 200 participants.

Duration of the Study

From January 2020 to March 2021

Data Collection

The survey was conducted in person, and later, due to COVID-19, online surveys were conducted through video conference and by email with the participants. – starting with senior officials and national level officials, followed by state level officials and then district and below.

Questions asked in the Survey

Questionnaire developed for the study is semi-structured with both the open-ended and close-ended questions being asked. The policy taken as a reference was the recently released National Health Policy in 2017.

The participants were asked (Close-ended)

1. If they were aware of the policy?
2. Have they read the policy?
3. Were they able to provide their inputs on the policy?
4. Awareness about the kind of studies used as evidence while formulating the policy.
5. Who were consulted while formulating the policy?
6. Their knowledge on the earlier health policies, and the implementation of policies.
7. The participants were asked if the health policy represented the healthcare problems/issues of their area, district, or state accurately.
8. The participants were asked if the policy addressed issues related to communicable diseases, non-communicable diseases, rare diseases, urban-rural divide, human resources and training, planning and programs, technology, administration and governance issues related to healthcare delivery, financing of health care, monitoring, and evaluation, the Make in India initiative, public-private partnerships, quality of health care, prevention, primary care, affordability, accessibility, needs of the tribals, needs of the hilly areas, needs of backward districts, malnutrition, senior citizens, and children.
9. The participants were asked about the role of various health care professionals including paramedics (nurses, pharmacists, physiotherapists, etc.), AYUSH professionals, etc in healthcare delivery.
10. The participants' opinion was sought on the competency of the paramedic professionals graduating from private institutions and did the National Health Policy 2017 address this issue.
11. The participants were asked if a separate health cadre, on the lines of IAS (Indian Administrative Service) and the IPS (Indian Police Service) is essential to manage the health care sector.

12. The participants were asked if the health policy addressed the issues about indigenous therapies such as AYUSH.
13. The participants were asked if monitoring and evaluation are important and if lack of time and accurate data, lack of technology driven systems, procedures and approvals required to share information, work overload, organizational silos, etc. were the key challenges in Monitoring &Evaluation (M&E).
14. The study subjects were asked to rate the quality of healthcare, and the quality of the available data on the health care.
15. They were asked if the NHP had an implementation framework and if its implementation brought about any changes in the health care system.
16. They were asked their opinion on the number of years after which the current NHP should be changed, and if every state should have its policy.
17. The participants were asked if healthcare should be the central, concurrent or a state subject.
18. The participants were asked if the National Council of Health and Family Welfare should meet once in three months, six months, or every year, or should it be dissolved.
19. The participants were asked to rank in order of influence on various stakeholders representing the right issues in the NHP-2017 between activists, NGOs, civil societies, or organizations, WHO, sustainable development goals, politicians, or patients.
20. The participants were asked to rank the issues (in order of influence) in the NHP-2017 between journalists, media, industry associations and bodies, CII, FICCI, ASSOCHAM, NATHEALTH, AHPI, private sector CEOs, prominent industry leaders, prominent doctors.
21. The participants were asked to rank representing the right issues (in order of influence) in the NHP-2017 between religious groups, bureaucrats, election manifesto, state officials, or paramedics or allied health care professionals.
22. The participants were surveyed about the extent of influence of different factors such as election manifesto, financial sustainability, donor funding, India's commitment to SDGs, availability of technology, new legislation, private-public partnerships, inter-sectoral coordination between ministries, private sector, academia, researchers, donors, evidence suggesting a reduction of disease burden due to certain health interventions in planning and decision making of the NHP- 2017.

23. The participants were asked about the extent of influence of different factors such as (human resources shortage, technical and technological resources, legal and regulatory challenges, frequent transfer of officials, financial challenges, medical supplies (demand and supply), inter-sectoral coordination between ministries, industry, academia, NGOs, researchers and donors, political championing by government officials, key stakeholders, communication and dissemination of information), on the implementation of the NHP- 2017.
24. The participants were asked if the NHP- 2017 addressed the following issues: communication and dissemination, human resources shortfall, technical-technological resources, legal and regulatory reform, frequent transfer of officials, financial challenges, medical supplies (demand and supply), inter-sectoral coordination between ministries, industry, academia, NGOs, researchers and donors, political championing by government officials, and key stakeholders.
25. The participants were asked to rank key challenges affecting the implementation of the National Health Policy 2017 in order of their importance; lack of clarity on goals, human resources shortfall, work overload of healthcare workers, inadequate training of healthcare workers, lack of coordination-siloed working, lack of financial resources, programs disconnected from ground realities, bureaucratic red-tapism, and delayed decision making, no freedom to try innovations.
26. The participants were asked to define the importance of data on different factors such as planning for healthcare programs, delivering appropriate health interventions, improving healthcare delivery while planning and implementing the NHP.
27. The participants were asked to rate the importance of various healthcare professionals and their effect on health care delivery. The professionals rated were ASHA and ANMs, doctors, nurses, pharmacists, healthcare counsellors, AYUSH professionals, local unqualified practitioners/quacks.

Open-ended questions:

The objective of the study is to suggest reforms / improvements in the policymaking process, and this required asking specific questions on improving the various components of the policymaking process, and related issues. Open ended questions tend to challenge the respondents on thinking beyond the choices given, and hence, in all, ten questions were asked from all the subjects at the levels of: the centre, the state and the district. The questions are as follows:

- What can be done differently to improve upon the communication and dissemination of information with regards to healthcare policies and programs?
- What are your suggestions to change/improve the policy planning process?
- Your suggestions to improve Monitoring and Evaluation of NHP.
- Your suggestions on improving the implementation of the National Health Policy 2017?
- Which indicators should be used to measure the effectiveness of a National Health Policy?
- Your suggestion for improving the quality of data with regards to healthcare.
- Your suggestion for improving the quality of healthcare?
- Your suggestions to make healthcare transparent, outcome-driven, and accountable?
- Your suggestions to utilize the AYUSH professionals effectively.
- Your suggestions to effectively utilize the role of paramedics (nurses, pharmacists, physiotherapists, etc).

Statistical Analysis

The data collected through the study has been analysed using the R software version 4.1.0 and the Excel. Categorical variables are put in the form of frequency table. Chi-square test has been used to check the dependency amongst the categorical variables. The P-value less than or equal to 0.05 indicates significance.

Findings

As a semi-structured questionnaire was used, the results are presented as quantitative and qualitative both.

Quantitative Results

Demographic characteristics of the study sample

Table 6 depicts the summary of the sample's demographic data. The respondents represented every age group, but a higher number of participants had less than 5 years' experience (62 percent) (Figure 3), wanted their details to be kept confidential (45.5 percent) (Figure 4) and the respondents were spread across the states.

Table 6: Summary of demographic data

Variables	Sub-Category	Number of Participants (%)
Total Experience	Less than 5 years	124 (62%)
	Between 5 and 10 years	25 (12.5%)
	More than 10 but less than 15 years	18 (9%)
	Between 15 - 20 years	14 (7%)
	More than 20 years	19 (9.5%)
State/Province	Bihar	19 (9.5%)
	Chandigarh	01 (0.5%)
	Delhi	03 (1.5%)
	Gujarat	01 (0.5%)
	Haryana	11 (5.5%)
	Jharkhand	06 (3%)
	Karnataka	07 (3.5%)
	Kerala	15 (7.5%)
	Madhya Pradesh	04 (2%)
	Maharashtra	07 (3.5%)
	Nagaland	07 (3.5%)
	Odisha	10 (5%)
	Punjab	44 (22%)
	Rajasthan	07 (3.5%)
	Tripura	15 (7.5%)
	Uttar Pradesh	21 (10.5%)
	Uttarakhand	22 (11%)

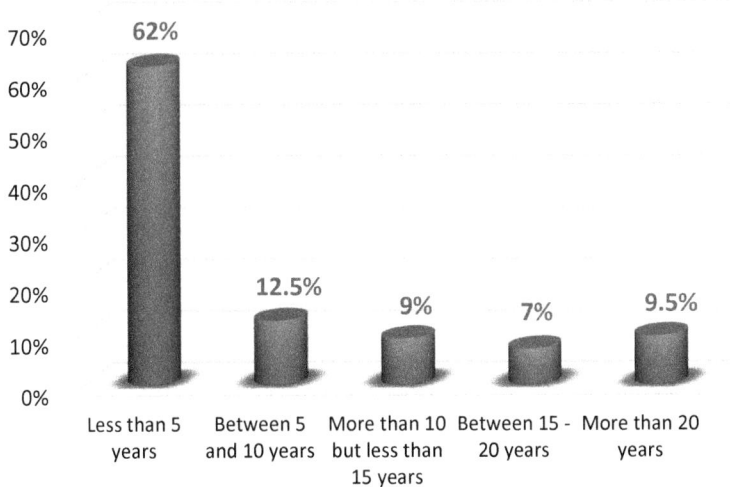

Figure 3: Distribution of participants according to their total experience

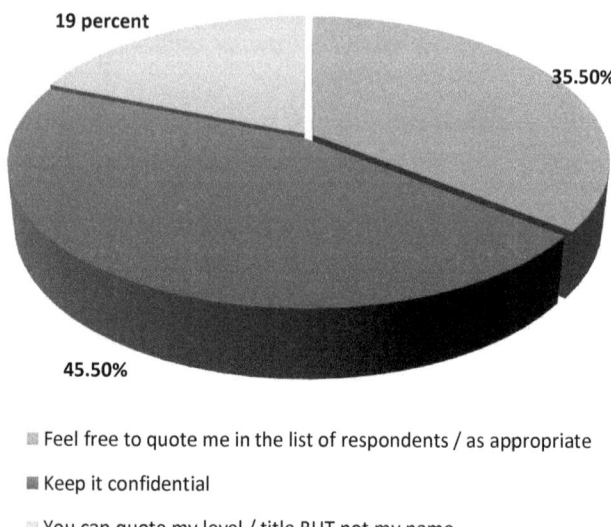

Figure 4: Distribution of participants according to acknowledging their participation in the study survey

Level of awareness on the NHP, 2017 among participants

Table 7 represents the responses of participants concerning the National Health Policy. Less than fifty percent of the participants had heard about the NHP, 2017, 42.5 percent had not read it, 36.5 percent had read it and 21 percent were not aware of it (Figure 5). Forty percent of participants were not aware that the policy was available in the public domain for inputs, while only 12 percent had provided their inputs (Figure 6). Forty-five percent of participants responded saying that the earlier health policies had been partially implemented and 27.5 percent of the respondents were not aware of the earlier health policies. (Figure 7).

Table 7: Awareness among participants about the National Health Policy- 2017

Variables	Sub-Category	Number of Participants (%)
With regards to the National Health Policy - 2017	I am not aware of the National Health Policy 2017	42 (21 %)
	I have heard about it but not read it	85 (42.5 %)
	I have read the National Health Policy	73 (36.5 %)
With regards to inputs to the NHP-2017	I know the policy was put in the public domain, but I could not share any inputs	71 (35.5 %)
	I am not aware that the policy was put in the public domain for inputs	80 (40 %)
	I could not find the link to the document in the public domain to share my inputs	25 (12.5 %)
	When the policy was put in the public domain, I gave my inputs	24 (12 %)
With regards to the earlier NHPs	I am not aware of the earlier health policies	55 (27.5 %)
	The earlier health policies have been implemented partially	90 (45 %)
	The earlier health policies have been implemented successfully	27 (13.5 %)
	The government failed to implement the earlier health policies	28 (14 %)

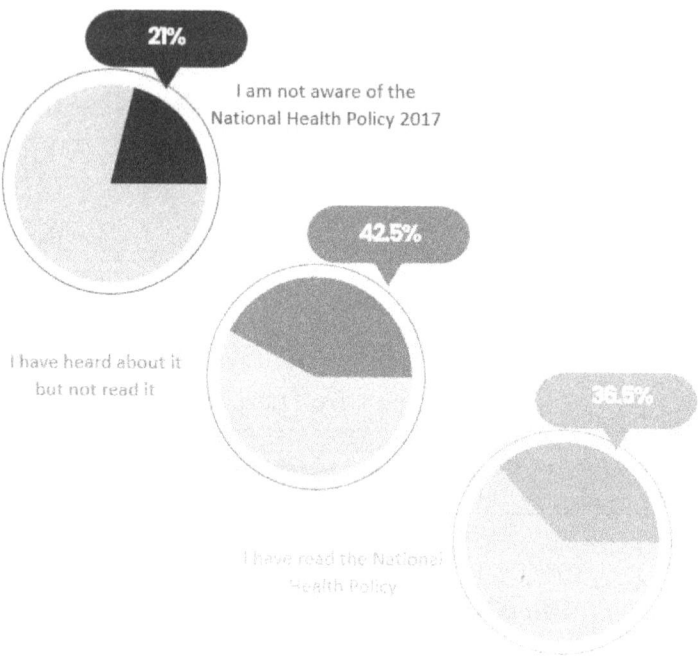

Figure 5: Awareness of the National Health Policy 2017

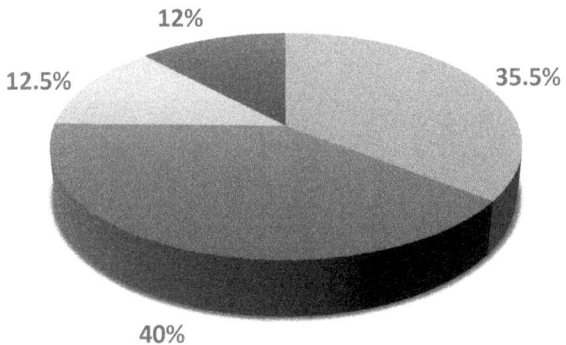

- I am aware of the fact that the policy was put in public domain, but i could not share any inputs
- I am not aware that the policy was put in public domain for inputs
- I could not find the link to the document in the public domain to share my inputs
- When the policy was put in public domain, i gave my inputs

Figure 6: Awareness on the provision to provide inputs to National Health Policy 2017

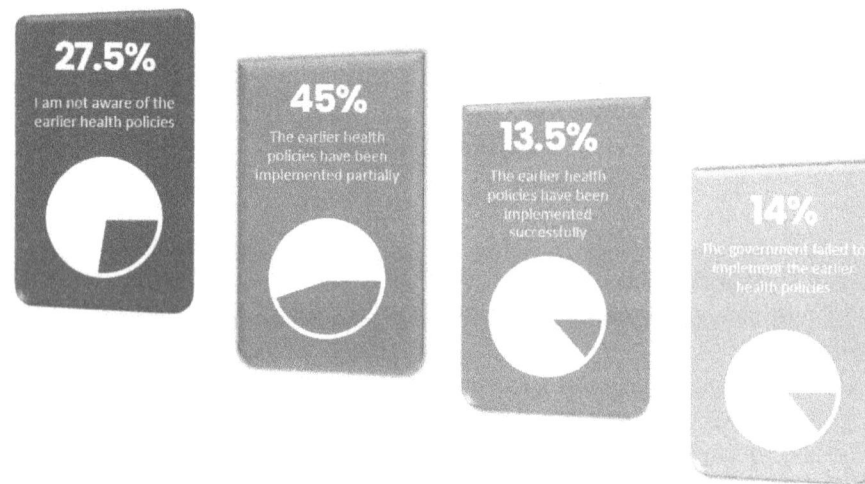

Figure 7: Awareness about the earlier National Health Policies

Perception of participants on the NHP, 2017

Table 8 presents the opinions of participants regarding various aspects of NHP-2017.

Majority of the respondents (37.5 percent) were not in a position to comment if the healthcare problems of their state, district or area were addressed. Only 6.5 percent of the respondents from semi-urban and the rural areas believed that healthcare problems in their area have been addressed, and only 7 percent of the respondents believed that the problems of their district have been addressed. 28 percent of the participants opined that the problems of their state were addressed by the NHP, 2017, while 10.5 percent opined that problems of their state were not addressed in the NHP, 2017 (Figure 8). 34 percent of participants felt that NHP is based on data from epidemiological studies, and only 16 percent believed that the NHP is backed by strong clinical evidence (Figure 9).

29 percent thought that the states were consulted for inputs with regards to the NHP-2017, whereas, 35 percent were not in the position to comment on the consultation process of the National Health Policy (Figure 10).

Table 8: Participant's opinions on various aspects of NHP- 2017

Variables	Sub-Category	Number of Participants (percent)
In your opinion, were the healthcare problems/issues of your area, district, or state accurately represented in the National Health Policy 2017?	Don't know. Can't Comment	75 (37.5 %)
	Problems of my area (semi-urban/ rural area) have been addressed	13 (6.5 %)
	Problems of my area (semi-urban/rural area) have NOT been addressed	14 (7 %)
	Problems of my district have been addressed	14 (7 %)
	Problems of my district have NOT been addressed	07 (3.5 5)
	Problems of my state have been addressed	56 (28 %)
	Problems of my state have NOT been addressed	21 (10.5 %)
In your assessment, with regards to the National Health Policy (NHP), which of the following applies	NHP is based on epidemiology studies	68 (34 %)
	NHP is not based on epidemiology studies	09 (4.5 %)
	NHP is backed by strong clinical evidence	32 (16 %)
	NHP is partly backed by evidence	28 (14 %)
	NHP is not backed by evidence	04 (2 %)
	Don't know. Can't comment	78 (39 %)
With regards to the National Health Policy 2017, which of the statements holds good?	States were consulted for inputs	58 (29 %)
	People working in the district level and below were consulted for inputs	57 (28.5 %)
	Consultations were only confined to the National level	30 (15 %)
	Don't know. Can't comment	70 (35 %)

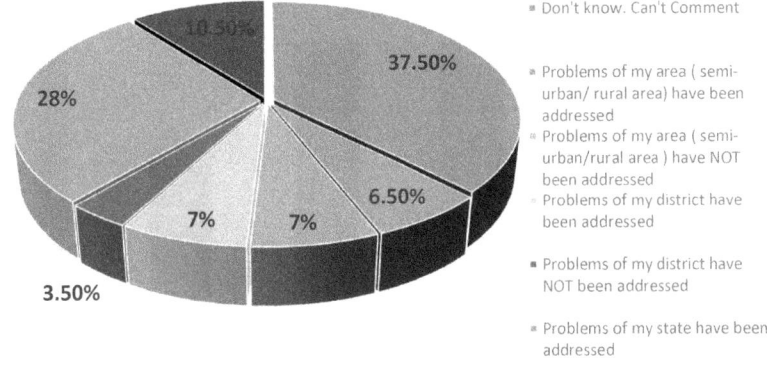

Figure 8: Opinions of participants when asked about healthcare problems/issues of their area, district, or state being accurately represented in the National Health Policy 2017.

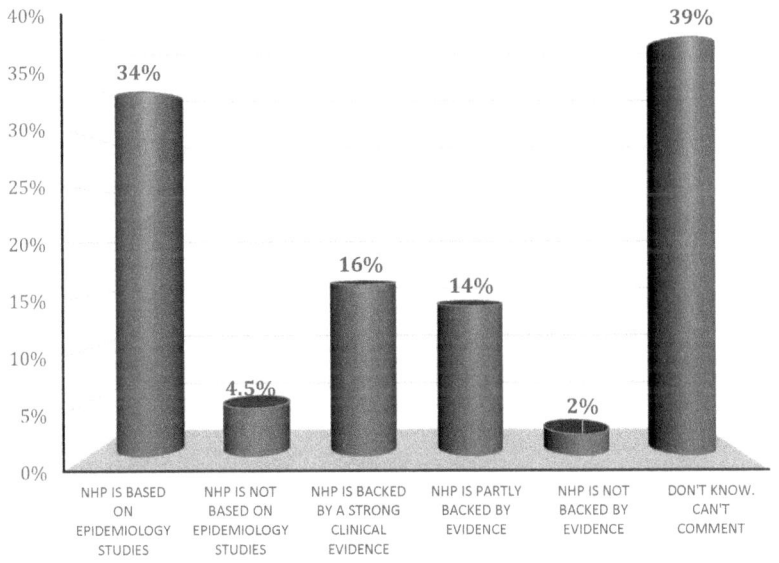

Figure 9: Opinions of participants on the data based on which NHP, 2017 was formulated.

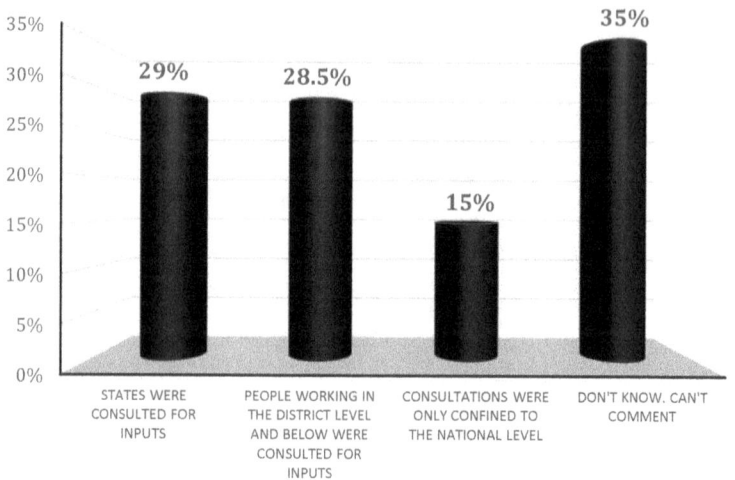

Figure 10: Participant's opinions on the individuals consulted while formulating the NHP, 2017

Issues addressed by NHP- 2017

Out of 200 participants, majority reported that NHP-2017 addressed communicable diseases (60.5 percent) and non-communicable diseases (53 percent). Less than half of the respondents believed that NHP, 2017 addressed; primary care (49.75 percent), planning and programming (47.72 percent), prevention (44.5 percent), children's health (43.5 percent), Affordability (40.5 percent), Malnutrition (39.5 percent), Quality of Care (39.5 percent), and healthcare of senior citizens (30.5 percent) (Table 9 and Figure 11).

The participants felt that needs of the tribals, backward class, and people from hilly areas were not addressed adequately. Rare diseases were another area of health that was opined to have been ignored in the NHP- 2017.

Table 9: Issues addressed by NHP- 2017 as opined by participants

Variables	Sub-Category	Number of Participants (percent)
Did the National Health Policy 2017 address the following? Check all that is applicable	Communicable diseases	121 (60.5 %)
	Non-communicable diseases	106 (53 %)
	Urban-rural divide	61 (30.5%)
	Human resources and training	90 (45 %)
	Planning and Programs	97 (48.5 %)
	Technology	58 (29 %)
	Administration and Governance issues related to healthcare delivery	74 (37 %)
	Financing of Healthcare	64 (32 %)
	Monitoring and Evaluation	64 (32 %)
	'Make in India' initiative	46 (23 %)
	Prevention	89 (44.5 %)
	Primary care	101 (50.5 %)
	Affordability	81 (40.5 %)
	Accessibility	79 (39.5 %)
	Needs of the Tribals	44 (22 %)
	Needs of hilly areas	41 (20.5 %)
	Needs of the most backward districts	51 (25.5 %)
	Malnutrition	79 (39.5 %)
	Public-Private Partnerships	64 (32 %)
	Quality of healthcare	79 (39.5 %)
	Senior citizens	61 (30.5%)
	Rare diseases	43 (21.5%)
	Children's health	87 (43.5%)

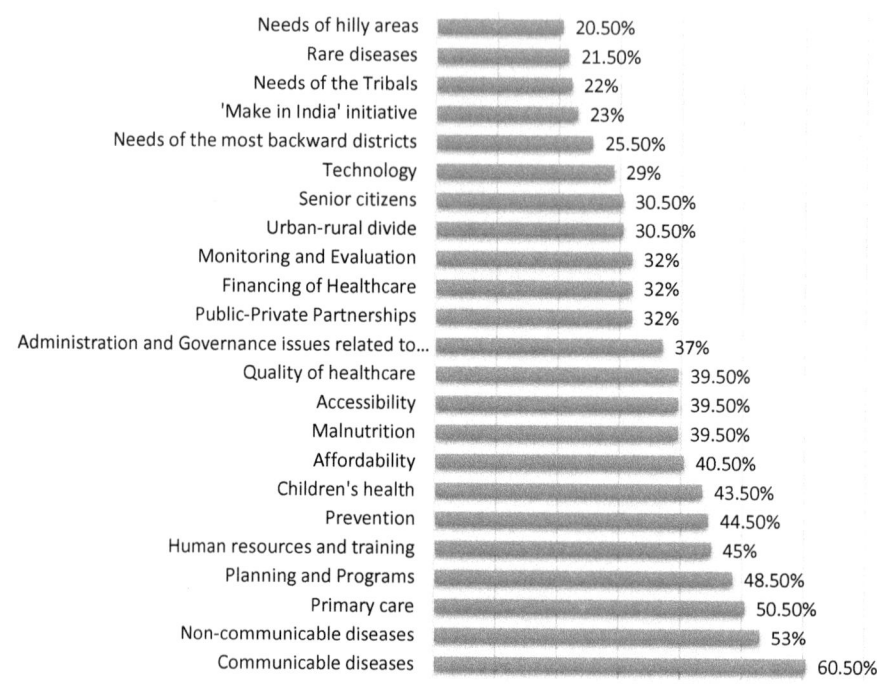

Figure 11: Issues addressed by NHP-2017 as opined by participants

Addressal of issues related to various Health care Professionals in NPH-2017

Of the total, 49.5 percent believed that NHP-2017 did a detailed analysis of the previous health policies and their impact on healthcare indicators (Figure 12). Sixty-four percent opined that paramedical staff (nurses, pharmacists, physiotherapists, etc.) were utilized effectively (Figure 13).

Of the respondents, 39.5 percent felt that the services of AYUSH professionals were effectively utilized in the Indian healthcare system (Figure 14).

81 percent thought that we need a separate cadre (dedicated cadre for healthcare service, like the other national services, on the lines of administrative, police services, etc.) (Figure 15).

65 percent opined that the National Health Policy-2017 addressed issues regarding indigenous therapies/AYUSH (Figure 16).

37 percent opined that the public sector institutions trained professionals with higher competence in comparison to professionals passing out of private institutions (Figure 17). According to 32 percent of participants, NHP-2017 addressed the issue of competence in medical, nursing, and allied health professionals coming out of the private institutions (Figure 18).

Table 10: Participant's opinions on addressing issues related to various health care professionals in NPH – 2017

Variables	Sub-Category	Number of Participants (percent)
Did the National Health Policy-2017 do a detailed analysis of the previous health policies and their impact on healthcare indicators?	Don't know. Can't comment	75 (37.5 %)
	No	26 (13 %)
	Yes	99 (49.5 %)
In your opinion, the role of paramedics (nurses, pharmacists, physiotherapists, etc.) has been utilized effectively	No	72 (36 %)
	Yes	128 (64 %)
Do you feel that the services of AYUSH professionals have been effectively utilized in Indian healthcare?	No	88 (44 %)
	No comments	33 (16.5 %)
	Yes	79 (39.5 %)
	No	38 (19 %)

Do you think we need a separate cadre (like the National Health Service on the lines of other national services akin to IAS, IPS, etc.) for healthcare	Yes	162 (81%)
Has the National Health Policy-2017 addressed the issues with regards to indigenous therapies /AYUSH?	No	70 (35 %)
	Yes	130 (65 %)
What is your assessment of the competence of medical, nursing, and allied health professionals coming out of the private institutions?	No comments	54 (27 %)
	No difference in competence levels	35 (17.5 %)
	The private sector churns out professionals with much better competence	37 (18.5 %)
	Public sector institutions churn out professionals with much better competence	74 (37 %)
Did the National Health Policy-2017 address the issue of competence of medical, nursing, and allied health professionals coming out of the private institutions?	No	61 (30.5 %)
	No comments	75 (37.5 %)
	Yes	64 (32 %)

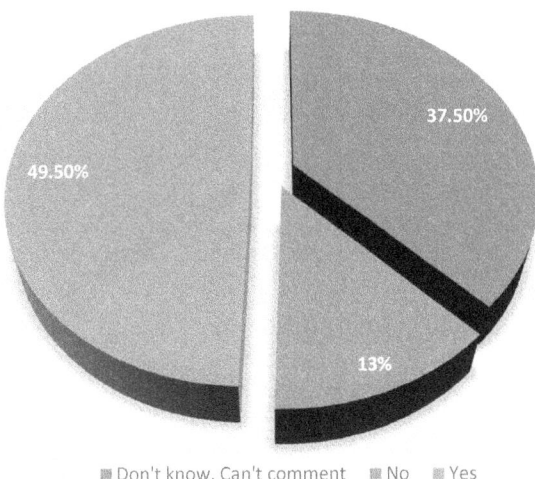

Figure 12: Participant's opinion on the formulation of NHP, 2017 after a detailed analysis of the previous health policies and their impact on various health care factors

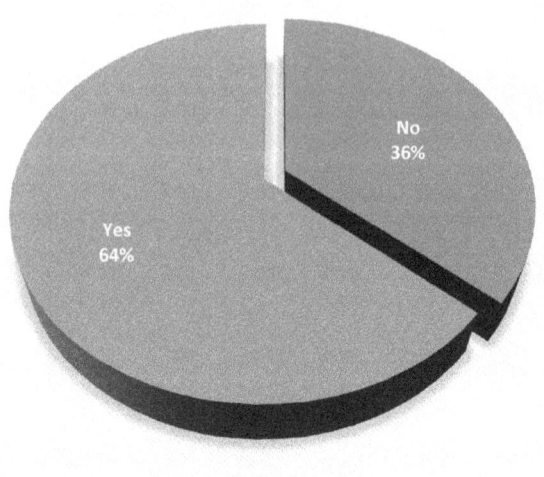

Figure 13: Participant's opinion about the role of paramedics (nurses, pharmacists, physiotherapists, etc.) being utilized effectively in the health care system

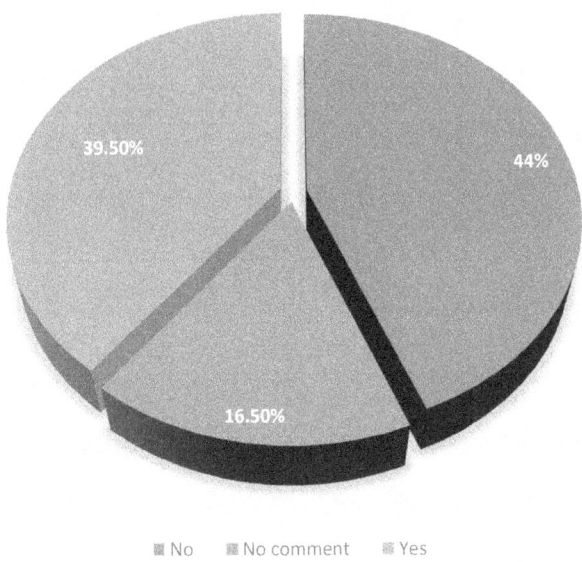

Figure 14: Opinion about the services of AYUSH professionals being effectively utilized in the Indian healthcare system

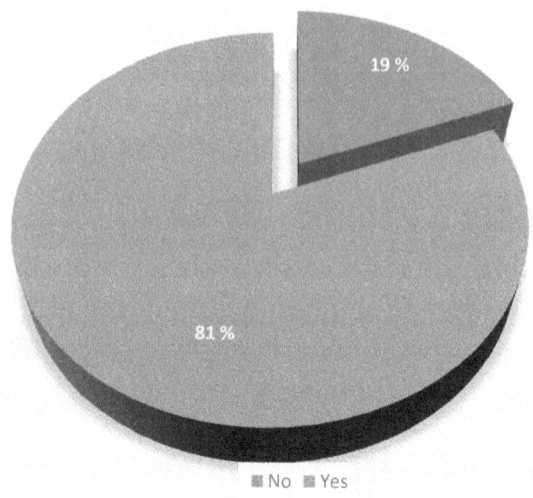

Figure 15: Opinion about the need for separate cadre (such as the National Health Service, on the lines of IAS, IPS, etc.) dedicated to health care

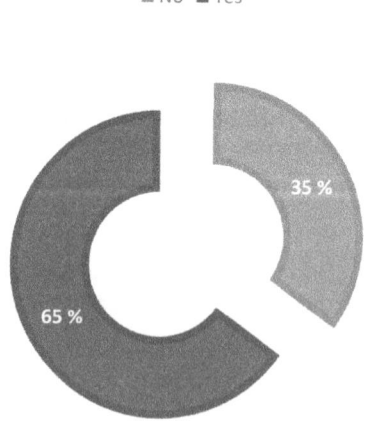

Figure 16: Opinion about National Health Policy 2017 addressing the issues with regards to indigenous therapies/AYUSH

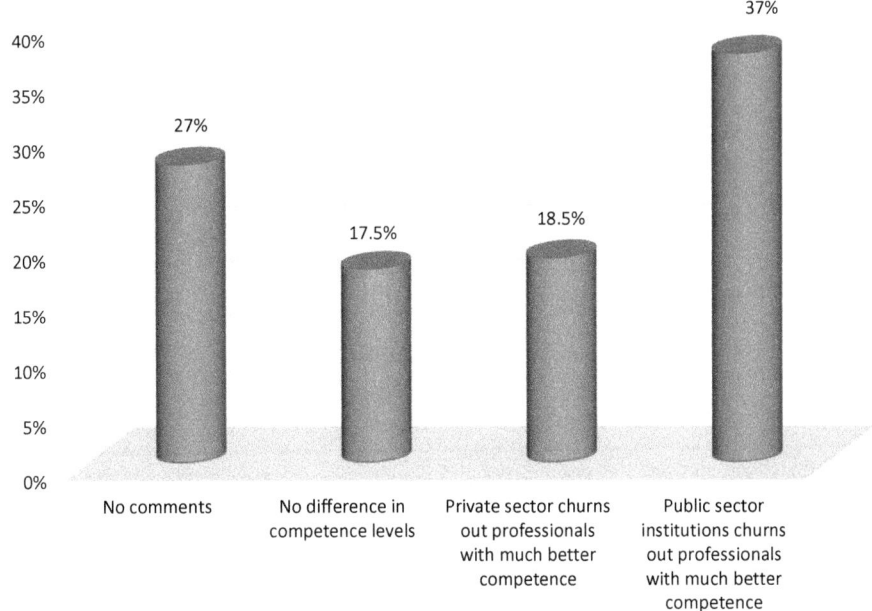

Figure 17: Opinion about the competence of medical, nursing, and allied health professionals coming out of private institutions

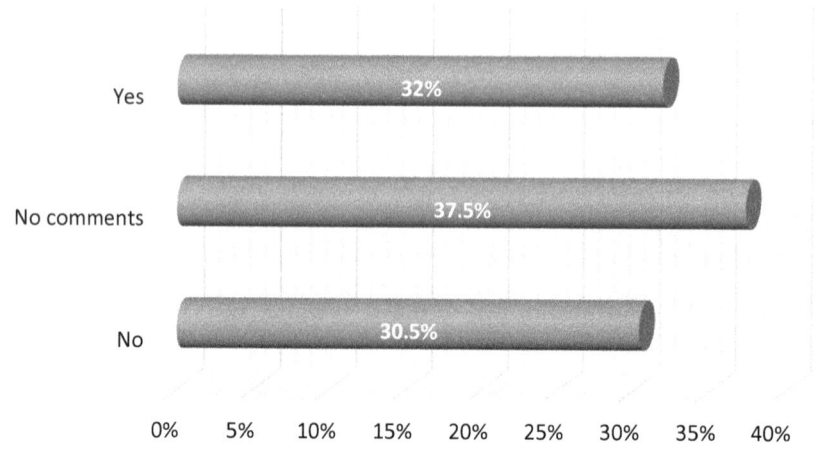

Figure 18: Opinion about the National Health Policy 2017 addressing the issue of competence in medical, nursing, and allied health professionals passing out of private institutions

Monitoring and Evaluation

The subjects studied had a good understanding of the significant role of monitoring and evaluation. 77 percent of participants opined that monitoring and evaluation are extremely important (Figure 19). The majority of participants shared that lack of timely and accurate data (63.5 percent), lack of technology-driven systems (53.5 percent), and procedures and approvals required to share information (46.5 percent), were the key challenges in monitoring and evaluation (Figure 20 and Table 11).

Table 11: Opinions of participants on Monitoring and Evaluation

Variables	Sub-Category	Number of Participants (percent)
In your opinion, how important are monitoring and evaluation?	Extremely important	154 (77 %)
	Not so important	06 (3 %)
	Somewhat important	40 (20 %)
What are the key challenges in Monitoring and Evaluation?	Lack of timely and accurate data	127 (63.5 %)
	Lack of Technology-driven systems	107 (53.5 %)
	Procedures and approvals needed to share information	93 (46.5 %)
	Siloed working	38 (19 %)
	Too much workload	71 (35.5 %)
	Others	18 (9 %)

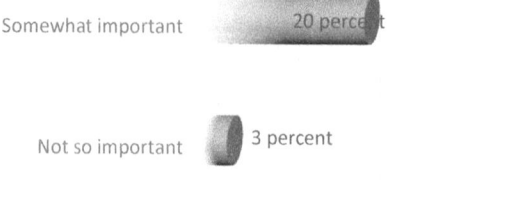
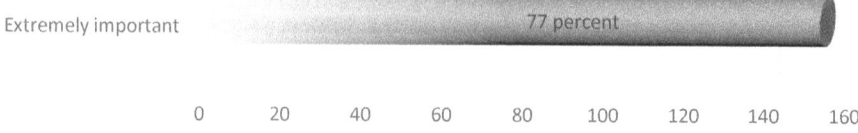

Figure 19: Importance of Monitoring and Evaluation

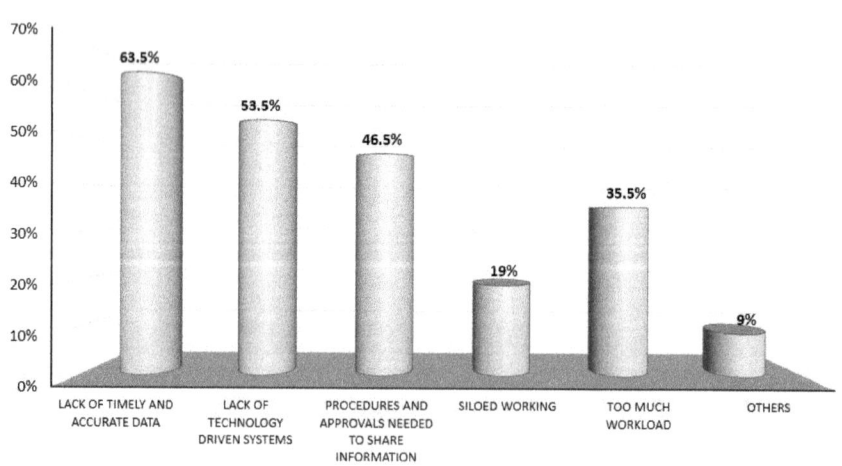

Figure 20: Key challenges in Monitoring and Evaluation

Quality of healthcare, healthcare data, healthcare policy, and suggestions for improvement

Table 12 represents the perception of participants on the quality of healthcare, healthcare data, healthcare policy, and suggestions for improvement.

Only a minuscule 7 percent rated the quality of services to be high. The quality of healthcare service in India was rated to be neither high nor low by 46.5 percent of participants (Figure 21).

When it comes to quality of data of healthcare, only 16 percent believe that the quality of data is high. A higher number of participants (61.5 percent) responded saying that the quality of data available with regards to healthcare in India is average (Figure 22).

A higher number of participants believed that NHP-2017 has an implementation framework (47.5 percent), and 37.5 percent were not aware of it and 15 percent didn't believe that the NHP-2017 has an implementation framework.

More than half (54.5 percent) of participants opined that NHP-2017 made a difference in healthcare.

When it comes to the time frame for drafting a new health policy, a higher number of participants believed that the National Health Policy-2017 should be drafted for 5 years (40.5 percent), and 25.5 percent want it to be drafted for 3 years, 18.5 percent for 10 years, 3 percent for 15 years and only 1.5 percent want it for 20 years. 11 percent stated that they want a long-term vision for healthcare factoring 25-50 years (Figure 23).

The majority of participants believe that every state should have its state health policy (67.5 percent) (Figure 24).

The National Council of Health and Family Welfare, which comprises of the union health minister, minister from states and other stakeholders, is the apex body for healthcare, as healthcare is a state subject. Of the total respondents, highest percentage (35.5 percent) believe it should meet every six months, 25.5 percent believe it should meet every three months and 16 percent believe it should meet every year and 7.5 percent of the respondents also believe that the Central Council has lost its relevance and it should be dissolved.

Table 12: Opinions of participants on quality of health care, healthcare data, health care policy, and changes suggested

Variables	Sub-Category	Number of Participants (percent)
How do you rate the quality of healthcare services in India?	High quality	14 (7 %)
	Low quality	40 (20 %)
	Neither high nor low quality	93 (46.5 %)
	Somewhat high quality	42 (21 %)
	Very low quality	11 (5.5 %)
How do you rate the quality of data about healthcare in India?	The average quality of data is available with regards to healthcare	123 (61.5 %)
	Data available is not at all trustworthy, and cannot be relied on for any level of decision making	45 (22.5 %)
	High quality of data is available with regards to healthcare	32 (16 %)
Did the National Health Policy-2017 have an implementation framework?	Don't know. Can't comment	75 (37.5 %)
	No	30 (15 %)
	Yes	95 (47.5 %)
Did the National Health Policy-2017 make a difference to healthcare?	Don't know. Can't comment	57 (28.5 %)
	No	34 (17 %)
	Yes	109 (54.5 %)
In your opinion, the National Health Policy - 2017 should be drafted for how many years?	10 years	37 (18.5 %)
	15 years	6 (3 %)
	20 years	3 (1.5 %)
	3 years	51 (25.5 %)
	5 years	81 (40.5 %)
	It should be for a longer-term vision for the country - the next 25 - 50 years	22 (11 %)
Should every state have its state health policy?	No	65 (32.5 %)
	Yes	135 (67.5 %)

Health should be	A Central (Union) Subject - The Parliament of India decides	54 (27 %)
	A Concurrent subject - both the Centre and state governments have the power to make laws. In case there is a conflict on the laws passed by Parliament and the state legislatures on the same subject, according to Constitution, the central law overrides the law framed by the state.	111 (55.5 %)
	Remain a state subject as it is now - Under this list, the state legislature may make the laws	35 (17.5 %)
How frequently should the National Council of Health and Family Welfare meet?	Every six months	71 (35.5 %)
	Every three months	51 (25.5 %)
	No comment	31 (15.5 %)
	Once a year	32 (16 %)
	The Central Council of Health & Family Welfare has lost its relevance and so, it should be dissolved	15 (7.5 %)

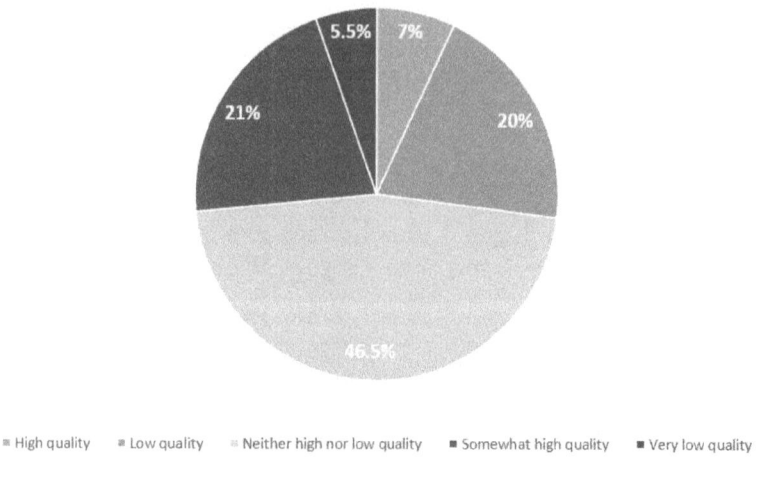

Figure 21: Rate the quality of healthcare services in India

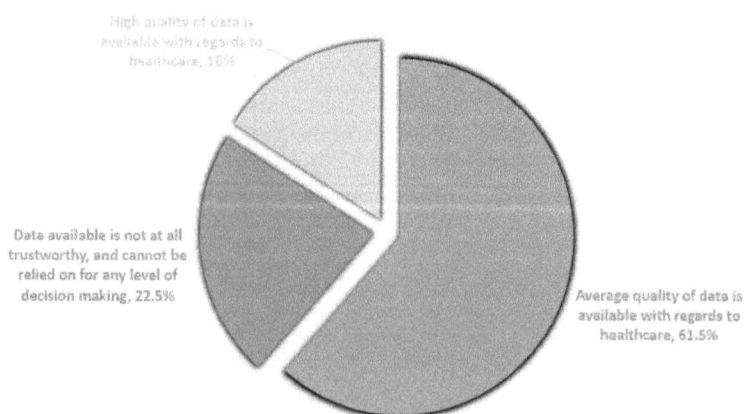

Figure 22: Quality of data with regards to healthcare in India

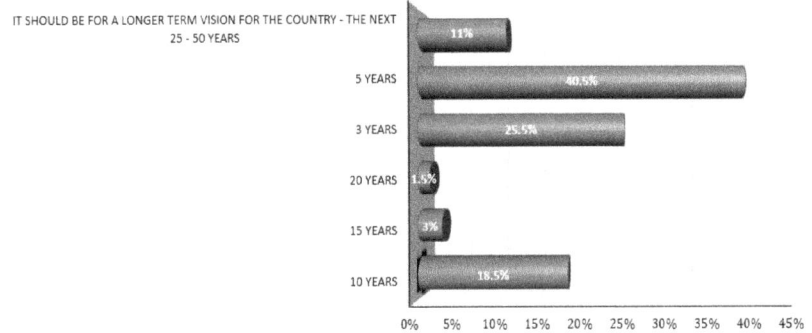

Figure 23: Opinion of participants on the number of years after which an NHP should be changed

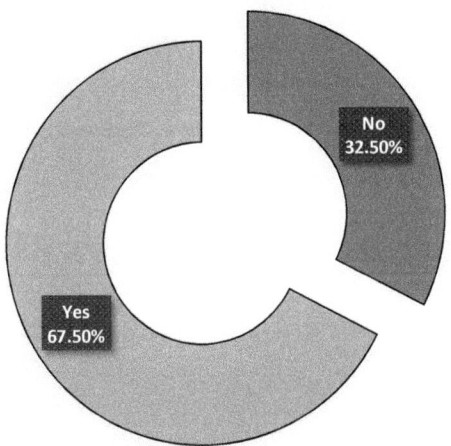

Figure 24: Opinion of participants about every state having its state health policy

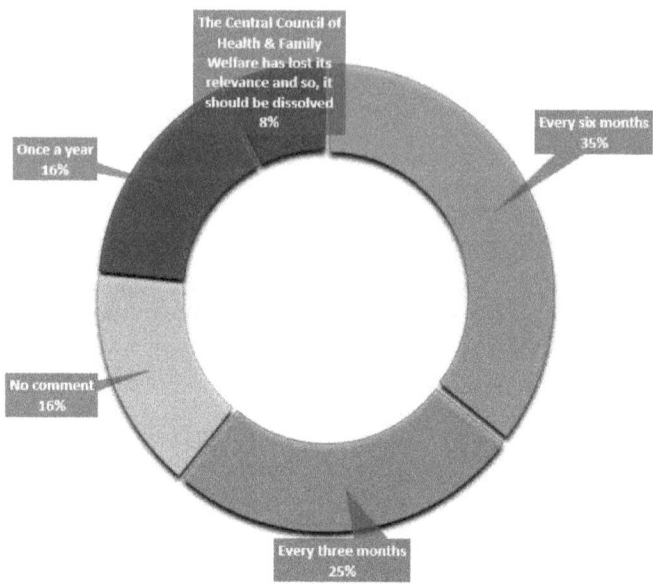

Figure 25: Opinion of participants about how frequently the National Council of Health and Family Welfare should meet

Table 12 (a): Association of opinion regarding NHP-2017 with total experience

Variables	Subcategory	Between 15 - 20 years	Between 5 and 10 years	less than 5 years	More than 10 but less than 15 years	More than 20 years	p-value
How do you rate the quality of healthcare services in India	High quality	0	2 (8%)	9 (7.26%)	1 (5.56%)	2 (10.53%)	0.1239^{MC}
	Low quality	6 (42.86%)	2 (8%)	21 (16.94%)	4 (22.22%)	7 (36.84%)	
	Neither high nor low quality	5 (35.71%)	10 (40%)	63 (50.81%)	8 (44.44%)	7 (36.84%)	
	Somewhat high quality	1 (7.14%)	8 (32%)	28 (22.58%)	3 (16.67%)	2 (10.53%)	
	Very low quality	2 (14.29%)	3 (12%)	3 (2.42%)	2 (11.11%)	1 (5.26%)	
How do you rate the quality of data with regards to healthcare in India?	Average quality of data is available with regards to healthcare	6 (42.86%)	14 (56%)	84 (67.74%)	6 (33.33%)	13 (68.42%)	0.0025^{MC}*
	Data available is not at all trustworthy, and cannot be relied on for any level of decision making	2 (14.29%)	7 (28%)	27 (21.77%)	4 (22.22%)	5 (26.32%)	
	High quality of data is available with regards to healthcare	6 (42.86%)	4 (16%)	13 (10.48%)	8 (44.44%)	1 (5.26%)	
Did the National Health Policy 2017 have an implementation framework?	Don't know. Can't comment	4 (28.57%)	10 (40%)	47 (37.9%)	7 (38.89%)	7 (36.84%)	0.7721^{MC}
	No	2 (14.29%)	2 (8%)	17 (13.71%)	5 (27.78%)	4 (21.05%)	
	Yes	8 (57.14%)	13 (52%)	60 (48.39%)	6 (33.33%)	8 (42.11%)	

Question	Answer						p-value
Did the National Health Policy 2017 make a difference to healthcare?	Don't know. Can't comment	1 (7.14%)	11 (44%)	32 (25.81%)	8 (44.44%)	5 (26.32%)	0.004^MC*
	No	2 (14.29%)	4 (16%)	16 (12.9%)	7 (38.89%)	5 (26.32%)	
	Yes	11 (78.57%)	10 (40%)	76 (61.29%)	3 (16.67%)	9 (47.37%)	
In your opinion, the National Health Policy 2017 should be drafted for how many years?	10 years	3 (21.43%)	6 (24%)	22 (17.74%)	4 (22.22%)	2 (10.53%)	0.9345^MC
	15 years	0	1 (4%)	4 (3.23%)	1 (5.56%)	0	
	20 years	0	0	3 (2.42%)	0	0	
	3 years	3 (21.43%)	6 (24%)	32 (25.81%)	4 (22.22%)	6 (31.58%)	
	5 years	6 (42.86%)	7 (28%)	50 (40.32%)	7 (38.89%)	11 (57.89%)	
	It should be for a longer-term vision for the country – the next 25 - 50 years	2 (14.29%)	5 (20%)	13 (10.48%)	2 (11.11%)	0	
Should every state have its own state health policy?	No	7 (50%)	6 (24%)	42 (33.87%)	6 (33.33%)	4 (21.05 percent)	0.4183^MC
	Yes	7 (50%)	19 (76%)	82 (66.13%)	12 (66.67%)	15 (78.95%)	
Health should be	A Central (Union) Subject - The Parliament of India decides	1 (7.14%)	5 (20%)	34 (27.42%)	7 (38.89%)	7 (36.84%)	0.1474^MC
	A Concurrent subject - both the Centre and state governments have the power to make laws. In case there is a	7 (50%)	16 (64%)	71 (57.26%)	7 (38.89%)	10 (52.63%)	

	conflict on the laws passed by Parliament and the state legislatures on the same subject, according to Constitution, the central law overrides the law framed by the state.					
	Remain a state subject as it is now - Under this list, the legislature of a state may make laws	6 (42.86%)	4 (16%)	19 (15.32%)	4 (22.22%)	2 (10.53%)	
How frequently should the National Council of Health & Family Welfare meet?	Every six months	3 (21.43%)	7 (28%)	49 (39.52%)	8 (44.44%)	4 (21.05%)	0.06[MC]
	Every three months	2 (14.29%)	10 (40%)	26 (20.97%)	4 (22.22%)	9 (47.37%)	
	No comment	4 (28.57%)	5 (20%)	20 (16.13%)	2 (11.11%)	0	
	Once a year	2 (14.29%)	1 (4%)	22 (17.74%)	4 (22.22%)	3 (15.79%)	
	The Central Council of Health & Family Welfare has lost its relevance and so, it should be dissolved	3 (21.43%)	2 (8%)	7 (5.65%)	0	3 (15.79%)	

Abbreviation: MC – Chi-square test with Monte Carlo simulation, * indicates statistical significance.

From Chi-square test, we observe that, opinion about the quality of data with regards to healthcare in India and whether the National Health Policy - 2017 did make a difference to healthcare, has significant association with total experience.

The following table gives association of opinion regarding NHP-2017 with designation.

Table 12 (b): Association of opinion regarding NHP-2017 with designation

Variables	Subcategory	Academician + Researcher	Civil Society Organization / NGO	Clinician	District level	National level	Private Sector	Semi-urban / rural area	State level	Others	p-value
How do you rate the quality of healthcare services in India	High quality	2 (6.67%)	0	2 (10.53%)	1 (5.26%)	2 (25%)	0	3 (10.71%)	2 (8%)	2 (3.85%)	0.004^MC*
	Low quality	7 (23.33%)	0	1 (5.26%)	1 (5.26%)	3 (37.5%)	3 (33.33%)	5 (17.86%)	7 (28%)	13 (25%)	
	Neither high nor low quality	15 (50%)	9 (90%)	6 (31.58%)	13 (68.42%)	2 (25%)	1 (11.11%)	17 (60.71%)	10 (40%)	20 (38.46%)	
	Somewhat high quality	3 (10%)	1 (10%)	5 (26.32%)	4 (21.05%)	1 (12.5%)	5 (55.56%)	3 (10.71%)	4 (16%)	16 (30.77%)	
	Very low quality	3 (10%)	0	5 (26.32%)	0	0	0	0	2 (8%)	1 (1.92%)	
How do you rate the quality of data with regards to healthcare in India?	Average quality of data is available with regards to healthcare	17 (56.67%)	7 (70%)	6 (31.58%)	9 (47.37%)	2 (25%)	2 (22.22%)	24 (85.71%)	15 (60%)	41 (78.85%)	< 0.001^MC*
	Data available is not at all trustworthy, and cannot be relied on for	11 (36.67%)	3 (30%)	5 (26.32%)	4 (21.05%)	4 (50%)	4 (44.44%)	4 (14.29%)	5 (20%)	5 (9.62%)	

117

	any level of decision making										p-value
High quality of data is available with regards to healthcare	2 (6.67%)	0	8 (42.11%)	6 (31.58%)	2 (25%)	3 (33.33%)	0	5 (20%)	6 (11.54%)	
Did the National Health Policy 2017 have an implementation framework?	Don't know. Can't comment	6 (20%)	6 (60%)	7 (36.84%)	10 (52.63%)	3 (37.5%)	6 (66.67%)	8 (28.57%)	4 (16%)	25 (48.08%)	<0.001^{MC*}
	No	9 (30%)	0	8 (42.11%)	0	2 (25%)	0	0	9 (36%)	2 (3.85%)	
	Yes	15 (50%)	4 (40%)	4 (21.05%)	9 (47.37%)	3 (37.5%)	3 (33.33%)	20 (71.43%)	12 (48%)	25 (48.08%)	
Did the National Health Policy 2017 make a difference to healthcare?	Don't know. Can't comment	4 (13.33%)	4 (40%)	4 (21.05%)	4 (21.05%)	2 (25%)	2 (22.22%)	10 (35.71%)	5 (20%)	22 (42.31%)	0.03998^{MC*}
	No	4 (13.33%)	0	7 (36.84%)	1 (5.26%)	3 (37.5%)	3 (33.33%)	4 (14.29%)	6 (24%)	6 (11.54%)	
	Yes	22 (73.33%)	6 (60%)	8 (42.11%)	14 (73.68%)	3 (37.5%)	4 (44.44%)	14 (50%)	14 (56%)	24 (46.15%)	
In your opinion, the National Health Policy 2017 should be	10 years	9 (30%)	0	7 (36.84%)	2 (10.53%)	2 (25%)	2 (22.22%)	4 (14.29%)	1 (4%)	10 (19.23%)	0.1454^{MC}
	15 years	3 (10%)	0	1 (5.26%)	0	0	1 (11.11%)	0	0	1 (1.92%)	

	20 years	3 years	5 years	It should be for a longer-term vision for the country - the next 25 - 50 years						MC
drafted for how many years?	0	8 (26.67%)	8 (26.67%)	2 (6.67%)						
		4 (40%)	6 (60%)	0						
		2 (10.53%)	7 (36.84%)	2 (10.53%)	4 (21.05%)	11 (57.89%)				
					1 (12.5%)	5 (62.5%)	0			
					3 (33.33%)	3 (33.33%)	0			
					10 (35.71%)	10 (35.71%)	4 (14.29%)			
	2 (8%)	9 (36%)	11 (44%)	2 (8%)						
	1 (1.92%)	10 (19.23%)	20 (38.46%)	10 (19.23%)						

	No	Yes		MC
Should every state have its own state health policy?	10 (33.33%)	20 (66.67%)		
	7 (70%)	3 (30%)		
	4 (21.05%)	15 (78.95%)		
	6 (31.58%)	13 (68.42%)		
	2 (25%)	6 (75%)		
	4 (44.44%)	5 (55.56%)		
	7 (25%)	21 (75%)		
	9 (36%)	16 (64%)		0.3153[MC]
	16 (30.77%)	36 (69.23%)		

	A Central (Union) Subject - The Parliament of India decides	A Concurrent subject - both the Centre and state governments	MC
Health should be	5 (16.67%)	20 (66.67%)	
	3 (30%)	5 (50%)	
	7 (36.84%)	6 (31.58%)	
	4 (21.05%)	9 (47.37%)	
	2 (25%)	5 (62.5%)	
	4 (44.44%)	4 (44.44%)	
	6 (21.43%)	19 (67.86%)	
	7 (28%)	13 (52%)	0.5727[MC]
	16 (30.77%)	30 (57.69%)	

have the power to make laws. In case there is a conflict on the laws passed by Parliament and the state legislatures on the same subject, according to Constitution, the central law overrides the law framed by the state. Remain a state subject as it is now - Under this list, the legislature of a state may make laws	5 (16.67%)	2 (20%)	6 (31.58%)	6 (31.58%)	1 (12.5%)	1 (11.11%)	3 (10.71%)	5 (20%)	6 (11.54%)	
How frequently should the National Council of Health & — Every six months	14 (46.67%)	2 (20%)	7 (36.84%)	4 (21.05%)	4 (50%)	1 (11.11%)	12 (42.86%)	9 (36%)	18 (34.62%)	0.2879^{MC}
Every three months	5 (16.67%)	4 (40%)	7 (36.84%)	4 (21.05%)	1 (12.5%)	2 (22.22%)	10 (35.71%)	6 (24%)	12 (23.08%)	

Family Welfare meet?									
No comment	4 (13.33%)	2 (20%)	2 (10.53%)	4 (21.05%)	2 (25%)	3 (33.33%)	4 (14.29%)	0	10 (19.23%)
Once a year	5 (16.67%)	2 (20%)	0	6 (31.58%)	1 (12.5%)	3 (33.33%)	1 (3.57%)	6 (24%)	8 (15.38%)
The Central Council of Health & Family Welfare has lost its relevance and so, it should be dissolved	2 (6.67%)	0	3 (15.79%)	1 (5.26%)	0	0	1 (3.57%)	4 (16%)	4 (7.69%)

*Abbreviation: MC – Chi square test with Monte Carlo simulation, * indicates statistical significance.*

From Chi-square test, we observe that, opinion of the respondents about; the quality of the healthcare data, whether National Health Policy 2017 has an implementation framework, and whether the National Health Policy 2017 did make a difference to healthcare, has significant association with designation.

Influence on representing the right issues at the NHP-2017

Influencers play key role in the policy formulation and Table 13 gives the rank in order of influence on representing the right issues in the National Health Policy 2017. A higher number of participants ranked; activists (31 percent) at 1, NGOs/Civil Society Organizations/Charities (29 percent) at 2, World Health Organization (18.5 percent) at 3, sustainable development goals (16 percent) at 4, politicians (17 percent) at 5 and patient groups (24 percent) at 6.

Table 13: Rank in order of influence on representing the right issues at the NHP 2017

(Column one gives the rank and rows against it give the number (percentage) of study respondents who rank it in that order).

Rank	Activists	NGOs / Civil Society Organizations / Charities	World Health Organization	Sustainable Development Goals	Politicians	Patient Groups
1	62 (31%)	18 (9%)	53 (26.5%)	23 (11.5%)	08 (4%)	09 (4.5%)
2	26 (13%)	58 (29%)	21 (10.5%)	32 (16%)	12 (6%)	08 (4%)
3	31 (15.5%)	30 (15%)	37 (18.5%)	27 (13.5%)	09 (4.5%)	09 (4.5%)
4	17 (8.5%)	30 (15%)	23 (11.5%)	32 (16%)	16 (8%)	14 (7%)
5	14 (7%)	12 (6%)	18 (9%)	26 (13%)	34 (17%)	11 (5.5%)
6	10 (5%)	20 (10%)	10 (5%)	16 (8%)	32 (16%)	48 (24%)
7	06 (3%)	11 (5.5%)	14 (7%)	08 (4%)	17 (8.5%)	28 (14%)
8	08 (4%)	04 (2%)	04 (2%)	12 (6%)	09 (4.5%)	22 (11%)
9	01 (0.5%)	05 (2.5%)	04 (2%)	05 (2.5%)	12 (6%)	05 (2.5%)

10	07 (3.5%)	02 (1%)	03 (1.5%)	05 (2.5%)	04 (2%)	09 (4.5%)
11	06 (3%)	03 (1.5%)	06 (3%)	04 (2%)	07 (3.5%)	11 (5.5%)
12	02 (1%)	02 (1%)	01 (0.5%)	06 (3%)	06 (3%)	07 (3.5%)
13	08 (4%)	00	02 (1%)	00	04 (2%)	07 (3.5%)
14	00	02 (1%)	00	02 (1%)	09 (4.5%)	04 (2%)
15	02 (1%)	03 (1.5%)	04 (2%)	02 (1%)	06 (3%)	05 (2.5%)
16	00	00	00	00	15 (7.5%)	03 (1.5%)

About the influencers representing the right issues in NHP-2017 as per the responses given by the participants (Table 14 and Table 15), around 22.5 percent have ranked journalists/media at 7, 17.5 percent have ranked industry associations and bodies like CII, FICCI, ASSOCHAM, NATHEALTH, AHPI at 8, 30.5 percent have ranked private sector CEOs at 9, 34 percent have ranked prominent industry leaders at 10, 31 percent have ranked Prominent doctors at 11 (Table 14). 36 percent of participants have ranked religious groups at 12, 38.5 percent have ranked bureaucrats at 13, 49 percent have ranked election manifesto at 14, 47 percent have ranked state officials at 15, 49 percent have ranked paramedics and allied health professionals at 16 (Table 15).

Table 14: Rank in order of influence on representing the right issues at the NHP 2017

(Column one gives the rank and rows against it give the number (percentage) of study respondents who rank it in that order).

Rank	Journalists / Media	Industry associations and bodies like CII, FICCI, ASSOCHAM, NATHEALTH, AHPI	Private Sector CEOs	Prominent Industry Leaders	Prominent doctors
1	03 (1.5%)	01 (0.5%)	03 (1.5%)	00	04 (2%)
2	09 (4.5%)	05 (2.5%)	04 (2%)	04 (2%)	04 (2%)
3	06 (3%)	19 (9.5%)	03 (1.5%)	02 (1%)	16 (8%)
4	08 (4%)	25 (12.5%)	06 (3%)	04 (2%)	12 (6%)
5	19 (9.5%)	19 (9.5%)	09 (4.5%)	04 (2%)	09 (4.5%)
6	19 (9.5%)	06 (3%)	05 (2.5%)	03 (1.5%)	11 (5.5%)
7	45 (22.5%)	23 (11.5%)	10 (5%)	08 (4%)	09 (4.5%)
8	29 (14.5%)	35 (17.5%)	25 (12.5%)	12 (6%)	07 (3.5%)
9	29 (14.5%)	27 (13.5%)	61 (30.5%)	18 (9%)	08 (4%)
10	10 (5%)	17 (8.5%)	23 (11.5%)	68 (34%)	22 (11%)
11	06 (3%)	07 (3.5%)	23 (11.5%)	33 (16.5%)	62 (31%)
12	03 (1.5%)	05 (2.5%)	11 (5.5%)	20 (10%)	26 (13%)
13	03 (1.5%)	08 (4%)	12 (6%)	12 (6%)	05 (2.5%)
14	01 (0.5%)	02 (1%)	01 (0.5%)	11 (5.5%)	03 (1.5%)
15	05 (2.5%)	01 (0.5%)	01 (0.5%)	01 (0.5%)	00
16	05 (2.5%)	00	03 (1.5%)	00	02 (1%)

Table 15: Rank in order of influence on representing the right issues at the NHP 2017

(Column one gives the rank and rows against it gives the number (percentage) of study respondents who rank it in that order).

Rank	Religious groups	Bureaucrats	Election Manifesto	State officials	Paramedics and allied health professionals
1	01 (0.5%)	04 (2%)	05 (2.5%)	03 (1.5%)	03 (1.5%)
2	01 (0.5%)	02 (%	02 (1%)	01 (0.5%)	11 (5.5%)
3	00	03 (1.5%)	00	03 (1.5%)	05 (2.5%)
4	01 (0.5%)	05 (2.5%)	01 (0.5%)	03 (1.5%)	03 (1.5%)
5	04 (2%)	01 (0.5%)	00	11 (5.5%)	09 (4.5%)
6	03 (1.5%)	03 (1.5%)	02 (1%)	07 (3.5%)	05 (2.5%)
7	01 (0.5%)	07 (3.5%)	02 (1%)	04 (2%)	07 (3.5%)
8	04 (2%)	08 (4%)	06 (3%)	05 (2.5%)	10 (5%)
9	06 (3%)	1(0.5%)	03 (1.5%)	11 (5.5%)	04 (2%)
10	07 (3.5%)	09 (4.5%)	04 (2%)	06 (3%)	04 (2%)
11	21 (10.5%)	08 (4%)	01 (0.5%)	02 (1%)	00
12	72 (36%)	26 (13%)	07 (3.5%)	03 (1.5%)	03 (1.5%)
13	30 (15%)	77 (38.5%)	11 (5.5%)	11 (5.5%)	10 (5%)
14	15 (7.5%)	27 (13.5%)	98 (49%)	11 (5.5%)	14 (7%)
15	11 (5.5%)	09 (4.5%)	42 (21%)	94 (47%)	14 (7%)
16	23 (11.5%)	10 (5%)	16 (8%)	25 (12.5%)	98 (49%)

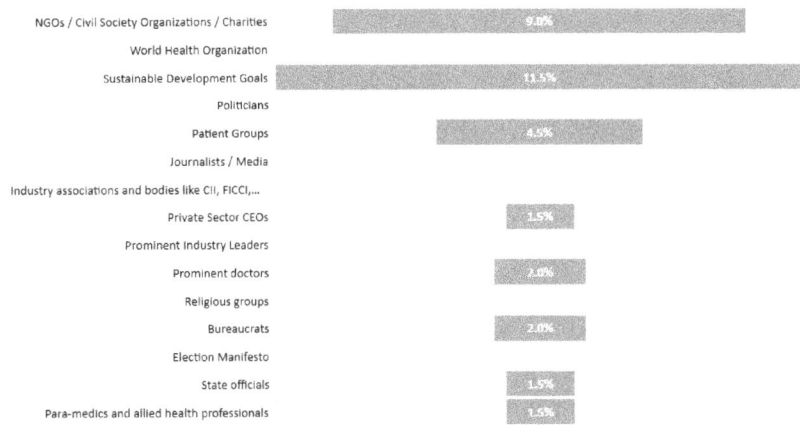

Order of influence on representing the right issues at the NHP-2017 (First Rank)

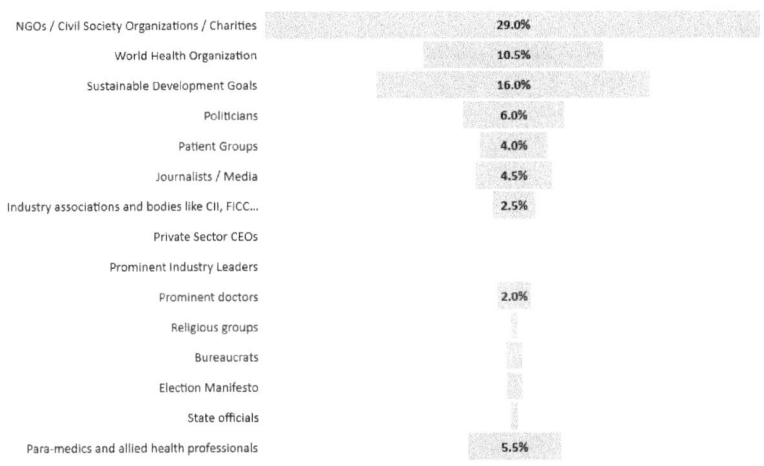

Order of influence on representing the right issues at the NHP-2017 (Second Rank)

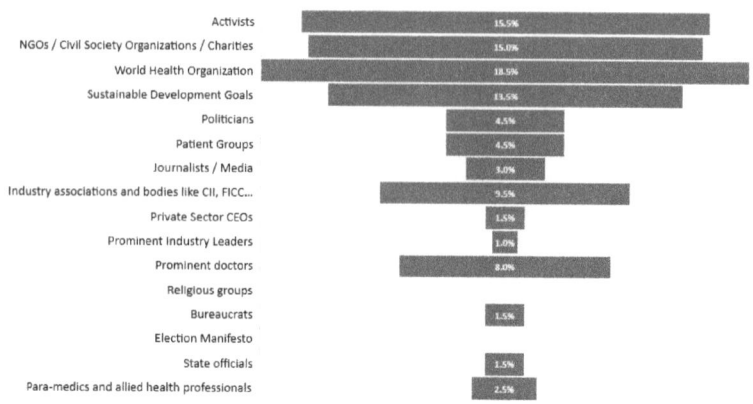

Order of influence on representing the right issues at the NHP-2017 (Third Rank)

Influence of different factors in the planning and decision making of the NHP-2017

Majority of the participants believed that all different factors including; election manifesto, financial sustainability, donor funding, India's commitment to SDGs, availability of technology, new legislation, private-public partnerships, inter-sectoral coordination between ministries, private sector, academia, researchers, donors, and evidence suggesting a reduction of disease burden due to certain health interventions, somewhat influenced the planning and decision making of the NHP-2017 (Table 16 and Figure 26).

When it comes to factors influencing the planning and decision making of the NHP-2017, availability of technology was rated the highest (32 percent), followed by the Election Manifesto (31 percent), followed by Financial sustainability and donor funding at 29 percent, followed by the evidence suggesting a reduction of disease burden due to certain health interventions at 27 percent, followed by India's commitment to SDGs (24 percent), donors (24 percent), inter-sectoral coordination between ministries (24 percent), Private Public Partnerships at 20 percent ,and new legislation at 14.5 percent.

Table 16: The extent of influence of different factors in the planning and decision making of the NHP-2017

Factors	Not much	Somewhat	To a large extent
Election Manifesto	20 (10%)	111 (55.5%)	62 (31%)
Financial Sustainability	15 (7.5%)	87 (43.5%)	58 (29%)
Donor funding	22 (11%)	77 (38.5%)	58 (29%)
India's commitment to SDGs	20 (10%)	83 (41.5%)	48 (24%)
Availability of Technology	9 (4.5%)	77 (38.5%)	64 (32%)
New legislation	21 (10.5%)	94 (47%)	29 (14.5%)
Private Public Partnerships	21 (10.5%)	79 (39.5%)	40 (20%)
Inter-sectoral coordination between ministries, private sector, academia, researchers, donors.	21 (10.5%)	68 (34%)	48 (24%)

| Evidence suggesting a reduction of disease burden due to certain health interventions | 14 (7%) | 70 (35%) | 54 (27%) |

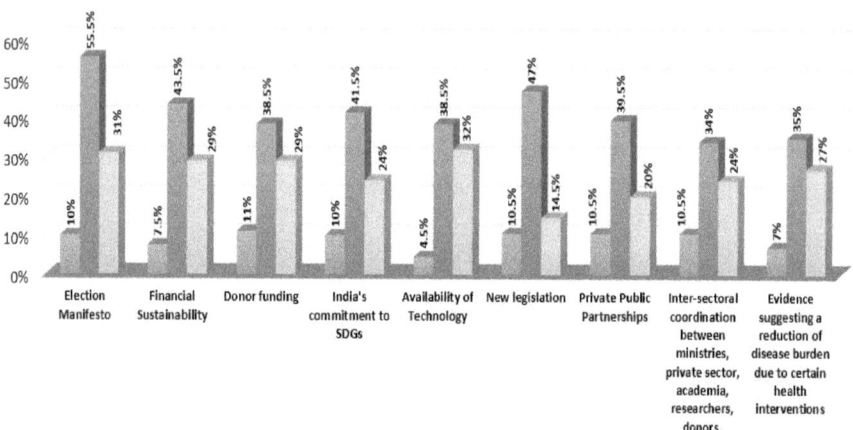

Figure 26: The extent of influence of different factors in the planning and decision making of the NHP-2017

The following table gives association of opinion about extent of influence of different factors on the planning and decision making of National Health Policy 2017 with total experience.

Table 16 (a): Association of opinion about extent of influence of different factors in the planning and decision making of the National Health Policy-2017 with total experience.

Variables	Subcategory	Between 15 - 20 years	Between 5 and 10 years	less than 5 years	More than 10 but less than 15 years	More than 20 years	p-value
Election Manifesto	Not much	2 (4.29%)	0	14 (11.29%)	1 (5.56%)	3 (15.79%)	0.6432^{MC}
	Somewhat	8 (57.14%)	14 (56%)	70 (56.45%)	12 (66.67%)	7 (36.84%)	
	To a large extent	4 (28.57%)	9 (36%)	37 (29.84%)	5 (27.78%)	7 (36.84%)	
Financial Sustainability	Not much	2 (14.29%)	1 (4%)	6 (4.84%)	4 (22.22%)	2 (10.53%)	0.0175^{MC}*
	Somewhat	7 (50%)	6 (24%)	59 (47.58%)	8 (44.44%)	7 (36.84%)	
	To a large extent	0	10 (40%)	41 (33.06%)	3 (16.67%)	4 (21.05%)	
Donor funding	Not much	3 (21.43%)	1 (4%)	11 (8.87%)	2 (11.11%)	5 (26.32%)	< 0.001^{MC}*
	Somewhat	6 (42.86%)	11 (44%)	46 (37.1%)	11 (61.11%)	3 (15.79%)	
	To a large extent	1 (7.14%)	4 (16%)	49 (39.52%)	0	4 (21.05%)	
India's commitment to SDGs	Not much	4 (28.57%)	3 (12%)	12 (9.68%)	1 (5.56%)	0	0.0185^{MC}*
	Somewhat	5 (35.71%)	8 (32%)	57 (45.97%)	9 (50%)	4 (21.05%)	
	To a large extent	0	5 (20%)	30 (24.19%)	5 (27.78%)	8 (42.11%)	
	Not much	2 (14.29%)	0	3 (2.42%)	2 (11.11%)	2 (10.53%)	0.006^{MC}*

Availability of Technology	Somewhat	6 (42.86%)	10 (40%)	46 (37.1%)	11 (61.11%)	4 (21.05%)	**0.0015^MC***
	To a large extent	1 (7.14%)	7 (28%)	48 (38.71%)	1 (5.56%)	7 (36.84%)	
New legislation	Not much	3 (21.43%)	2 (8%)	7 (5.65%)	5 (27.78%)	4 (21.05%)	
	Somewhat	5 (35.71%)	7 (28%)	69 (55.65%)	9 (50%)	4 (21.05%)	
	To a large extent	0	6 (24%)	21 (16.94%)	0	2 (10.53%)	
Private Public Partnerships	Not much	2 (14.29%)	4 (16%)	13 (10.48%)	0	2 (10.53%)	0.061^MC
	Somewhat	5 (35.71%)	5 (20%)	51 (41.13%)	10 (55.56%)	8 (42.11%)	
	To a large extent	0	7 (28%)	30 (24.19%)	3 (16.67%)	0	
Inter-sectoral coordination between ministries, private sector, academia, researchers, donors.	Not much	2 (14.29%)	7 (28%)	8 (6.45%)	1 (5.56%)	3 (15.79%)	**0.003^MC***
	Somewhat	5 (35.71%)	3 (12%)	50 (40.32%)	5 (27.78%)	5 (26.32%)	
	To a large extent	0	7 (28%)	32 (25.81%)	7 (38.89%)	2 (10.53%)	
Evidence suggesting a reduction of disease burden due to certain health interventions	Not much	0	3 (12%)	9 (7.26%)	0	2 (10.53%)	**0.02999^MC***
	Somewhat	5 (35.71%)	8 (32%)	41 (33.06%)	11 (61.11%)	5 (26.32%)	
	To a large extent	0	4 (16%)	45 (36.29%)	2 (11.11%)	3 (15.79%)	

Abbreviation: MC – Chi-square test with Monte Carlo simulation, * indicates statistical significance.

From the Chi-square test, we observe that, opinion about the extent of influence of Financial Sustainability, Donor funding, India's commitment to SDGs, Availability of Technology, New legislation, Inter-sectoral coordination between ministries, private sector, academia, researchers, donors and evidence suggesting a reduction of disease burden due to certain health interventions in planning and decision making of National Health Policy-2017, has a significant association with the total experience.

The following table gives an association of opinion about the extent of influence of different factors in planning and decision making of National Health Policy-2017 with designation.

Table 16 (b): Association of opinion about extent of influence of different factors in the planning and decision making of the National Health Policy 2017 with designation.

Variables	Subcategory	Academician + Researcher	Civil Society Organization / NGO	Clinician	District level	National level	Private Sector	Semi-urban / rural area	State level	Others	p-value
Election Manifesto	Not much	5 (16.67%)	0	0	3 (15.79%)	2 (25%)	0	1 (3.57%)	1 (4%)	8 (15.38%)	0.1099^MC
	Somewhat	13 (43.33%)	10 (100%)	11 (57.89%)	9 (47.37%)	2 (25%)	5 (55.56%)	18 (64.29%)	16 (64%)	27 (51.92%)	
	To a large extent	12 (40%)	0	5 (26.32%)	7 (36.84%)	4 (50%)	4 (44.44%)	9 (32.14%)	7 (28%)	14 (26.92%)	
Financial Sustainability	Not much	2 (6.67%)	2 (20%)	0 (0%)	2 (10.53%)	1 (12.5%)	0	4 (14.29%)	3 (12%)	1 (1.92%)	0.068^MC
	Somewhat	15 (50%)	5 (50%)	9 (47.37%)	3 (15.79%)	3 (37.5%)	6 (66.67%)	12 (42.86%)	10 (40%)	24 (46.15%)	

	To a large extent	13 (43.33%)	0	4 (21.05%)	9 (47.37%)	3 (37.5%)	0	8 (28.57%)	5 (20%)	16 (30.77%)	
Donor funding	Not much	3 (10%)	2 (20%)	1 (5.26%)	2 (10.53%)	2 (25%)	4 (44.44%)	1 (3.57%)	1 (4%)	6 (11.54%)	**0.002**^{MC}*
	Somewhat	8 (26.67%)	3 (30%)	8 (42.11%)	7 (36.84%)	3 (37.5%)	2 (22.22%)	10 (35.71%)	10 (40%)	26 (50%)	
	To a large extent	17 (56.67%)	2 (20%)	4 (21.05%)	5 (26.32%)	2 (25%)	0	13 (46.43%)	7 (28%)	8 (15.38%)	
India's commitment to SDGs	Not much	4 (13.33%)	0	1 (5.26%)	2 (10.53%)	1 (12.5%)	1 (11.11%)	3 (10.71%)	1 (4%)	7 (13.46%)	0.9505^{MC}
	Somewhat	13 (43.33%)	5 (50%)	6 (31.58%)	7 (36.84%)	5 (62.5%)	3 (33.33%)	15 (53.57%)	9 (36%)	20 (38.46%)	
	To a large extent	11 (36.67%)	2 (20%)	3 (15.79%)	5 (26.32%)	1 (12.5%)	2 (22.22%)	4 (14.29%)	8 (32%)	12 (23.08%)	
Availability of Technology	Not much	0	0	0	3 (15.79%)	0	1 (11.11%)	0	1 (4%)	4 (7.69%)	0.1154^{MC}
	Somewhat	15 (50%)	5 (50%)	4 (21.05%)	6 (31.58%)	4 (50%)	5 (55.56%)	8 (28.57%)	10 (40%)	20 (38.46%)	
	To a large extent	13 (43.33%)	0	9 (47.37%)	5 (26.32%)	3 (37.5%)	1 (11.11%)	10 (35.71%)	7 (28%)	16 (30.77%)	

New legislation	Not much	4 (13.33%)	2 (20%)	0	3 (15.79%)	2 (25%)	2 (22.22%)	3 (10.71%)	2 (8%)	3 (5.77%)	0.3538[MC]
	Somewhat	20 (66.67%)	3 (30%)	8 (42.11%)	8 (42.11%)	5 (62.5%)	4 (44.44%)	8 (28.57%)	12 (48%)	26 (50%)	
	To a large extent	3 (10%)	0	4 (21.05%)	3 (15.79%)	0	1 (11.11%)	7 (25%)	3 (12%)	8 (15.38%)	
Private Public Partnerships	Not much	3 (10%)	0	2 (10.53%)	4 (21.05%)	1 (12.5%)	1 (11.11%)	6 (21.43%)	1 (4%)	3 (5.77%)	0.3118[MC]
	Somewhat	16 (53.33%)	3 (30%)	6 (31.58%)	4 (21.05%)	3 (37.5%)	4 (44.44%)	12 (42.86%)	9 (36%)	22 (42.31%)	
	To a large extent	8 (26.67%)	0	4 (21.05%)	6 (31.58%)	3 (37.5%)	0	2 (7.14%)	5 (20%)	12 (23.08%)	
Inter-sectoral coordination between ministries, private sector, academia, researchers, donors.	Not much	2 (6.67%)	0	2 (10.53%)	3 (15.79%)	1 (12.5%)	2 (22.22%)	5 (17.86%)	1 (4%)	5 (9.62%)	0.6452[MC]
	Somewhat	13 (43.33%)	1 (10%)	7 (36.84%)	5 (26.32%)	3 (37.5%)	2 (22.22%)	7 (25%)	7 (28%)	23 (44.23%)	
	To a large extent	12 (40%)	2 (20%)	5 (26.32%)	4 (21.05%)	3 (37.5%)	1 (11.11%)	6 (21.43%)	7 (28%)	8 (15.38%)	

Evidence suggesting a reduction of disease burden due to certain health interventions										p-value
Not much	2 (6.67%)	0	0	0	0	1 (11.11%)	3 (10.71%)	2 (8%)	6 (11.54%)	0.05997^MC
Somewhat	8 (26.67%)	3 (30%)	7 (36.84%)	6 (31.58%)	3 (37.5%)	4 (44.44%)	13 (46.43%)	5 (20%)	21 (40.38%)	
To a large extent	17 (56.67%)	0	5 (26.32%)	6 (31.58%)	4 (50%)	0	4 (14.29%)	8 (32%)	10 (19.23%)	

Abbreviation: MC – Chi-square test with Monte Carlo simulation, * indicates statistical significance.

From the Chi-square test, we observe that opinion about the extent of influence of Donor funding in planning and decision making of National Health Policy-2017, has a significant association with designation.

The majority of participants believed that human resources shortage (47.5%), financial challenges (42.5%), medical supplies (demand and supply) (35%), and communication and dissemination of information (46%), influenced the implementation of National Health Policy 2017 to large extent. Furthermore, majority of the participants believed that technical and technological resources (43.5 percent), legal and regulatory challenges (47 percent), frequent transfer of officials (49.5 percent), inter-sectoral coordination between ministries, industry, academia, NGOs, researchers, and donors (38.5 percent), political championing by government officials (33.5 percent) and key stakeholders (39.5 percent), influenced the implementation of the NHP-2017 to some extent (Table 17 and Figure 27).

Table 17: The extent of influence of different factors in the implementation of NHP 2017

Factors	Not much	Somewhat	To a large extent
Human Resources shortage	13 (6.5%)	82 (41%)	95 (47.5%)
Technical and Technological resources	09 (4.5%)	87 (43.5%)	62 (31%)
Legal and regulatory challenges	18 (9%)	94 (47%)	39 (19.5%)
Frequent transfer of officials	24 (12%)	99 (49.5%)	26 (13%)
Financial challenges	09 (4.5%)	49 (24.5%)	85 (42.5%)
Medical supplies (demand and supply)	09 (4.5%)	65 (32.5%)	70 (35%)
Inter-sectoral coordination between ministries, industry, academia, NGOs, researchers, and donors	11 (5.5%)	77 (38.5%)	50 (25%)
Political championing by Government officials	16 (8%)	67 (33.5%)	55 (27.5%)
Key stakeholders	18 (9%)	79 (39.5%)	34 (17%)
Communication and dissemination of information	23 (11.5%)	85 (42.5%)	92 (46%)

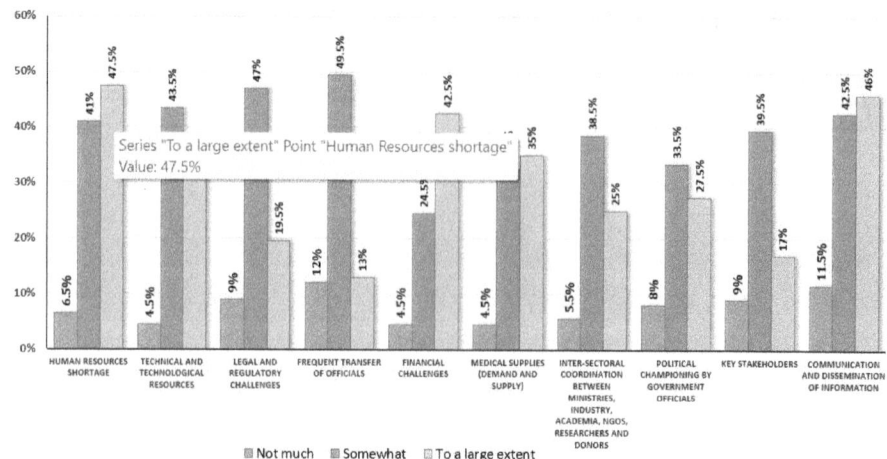

Figure 27: The extent of influence of different factors in the implementation of the NHP-2017

The following table gives association of opinion about extent of influence of different factors in implementation of the NHP-2017 with total experience.

Table 17 (a): Association of opinion about extent of influence of different factors in implementation of the NHP- 2017 with total experience.

Variables	Subcategory	Between 15 - 20 years	Between 5 and 10 years	less than 5 years	More than 10 but less than 15 years	More than 20 years	p-value
Human Resources shortage	Not much	0	1 (4%)	10 (8.06%)	0	2 (10.53%)	0.4523^{MC}
	Somewhat	9 (64.29%)	7 (28%)	53 (42.74%)	6 (33.33%)	7 (36.84%)	
	To a large extent	5 (35.71%)	15 (60%)	56 (45.16%)	9 (50%)	10 (52.63%)	
Technical and Technological resources	Not much	0	0	7 (5.65%)	0	2 (10.53%)	0.2614^{MC}
	Somewhat	6 (42.86%)	9 (36%)	60 (48.39%)	8 (44.44%)	4 (21.05%)	
	To a large extent	5 (35.71%)	10 (40%)	34 (27.42%)	5 (27.78%)	8 (42.11%)	
Legal and regulatory challenges	Not much	0	0	16 (12.9%)	1 (5.56%)	1 (5.26%)	0.2884^{MC}
	Somewhat	6 (42.85%)	9 (36%)	64 (51.61%)	9 (50%)	6 (31.58%)	
	To a large extent	3 (21.43%)	7 (28%)	21 (16.94%)	3 (16.67%)	5 (26.32%)	
Frequent transfer of officials	Not much	1 (7.14%)	4 (16%)	16 (12.9%)	2 (11.11%)	1 (5.26%)	0.9405^{MC}
	Somewhat	5 (35.71%)	11 (44%)	65 (52.42%)	10 (55.56%)	8 (42.11%)	
	To a large extent	2 (14.29%)	2 (8%)	18 (14.52%)	1 (5.56%)	3 (15.79%)	
Financial challenges	Not much	0	4 (16%)	4 (3.23%)	(0%)	1 (5.26%)	0.086^{MC}
	Somewhat	3 (21.43%)	3 (12%)	33 (26.61%)	7 (38.89%)	3 (15.79%)	
	To a large extent	4 (28.57%)	10 (40%)	57 (45.97%)	6 (33.33%)	8 (42.11%)	

Factor	Level						p-value
Medical supplies (demand and supply)	Not much	1 (7.14%)	4 (16%)	4 (3.23%)		0	0.0065^{MC}*
	Somewhat	5 (35.71%)	2 (8%)	44 (35.48%)	10 (55.56%)	4 (21.05%)	
	To a large extent	1 (7.14%)	12 (48%)	48 (38.71%)	4 (22.22%)	5 (26.32%)	
Inter-sectoral coordination between ministries, industry, academia, NGOs, researchers, and donors	Not much	1 (7.14%)	1 (4%)	8 (6.45%)	0	1 (5.26%)	0.2774^{MC}
	Somewhat	3 (21.43%)	8 (32%)	49 (39.52%)	13 (72.22%)	4 (21.05%)	
	To a large extent	2 (14.29%)	7 (28%)	36 (29.03%)	1 (5.56%)	4 (21.05%)	
Political championing by Government officials	Not much	1 (7.14%)	0	13 (10.48%)	2 (11.11%)	0	0.1099^{MC}
	Somewhat	1 (7.14%)	5 (20%)	48 (38.71%)	6 (33.33%)	7 (36.84%)	
	To a large extent	2 (14.29%)	12 (48%)	34 (27.42%)	5 (27.78%)	2 (10.53%)	
Key stakeholders	Not much	2 (14.29%)	3 (12%)	10 (8.06%)	2 (11.11%)	1 (5.26%)	0.1054^{MC}
	Somewhat	0	11 (44%)	57 (45.97%)	7 (38.89%)	4 (21.05%)	
	To a large extent	2 (14.29%)	1 (4%)	25 (20.16%)	2 (11.11%)	4 (21.05%)	
Communication and dissemination of information	Not much	4 (28.57%)	4 (16%)	7 (5.65%)	5 (27.78%)	3 (15.79%)	0.0485^{MC}*
	Somewhat	6 (42.86%)	10 (40%)	58 (46.77%)	5 (27.78%)	6 (31.58%)	
	To a large extent	4 (28.57%)	11 (44%)	59 (47.58%)	8 (44.44%)	10 (52.63%)	

Abbreviation: MC – Chi-square test with Monte Carlo simulation, * indicates statistical significance.

From Chi-square test, we observe that, opinion about extent of influence of medical supplies (demand and supply) and Communication and dissemination of information in implementation of the NHP-2017, has significant association with total experience.

The following table gives association of opinion about extent of influence of different factors in implementation of the NHP-2017 with designation.

Table 17 (b): Association of opinion about extent of influence of different factors in implementation of the NHP-2017 with designation.

Variables	Subcategory	Academician+ Researcher	Civil Society Organization /NGO	Clinician	District level	National level	Private Sector	Semi - urban / rural area	State level	Others	p-value
Human Resources shortage	Not much	0	0	3 (15.79%)	0	0	0	5 (17.86%)	1 (4%)	4 (7.69%)	**0.0405** MC*
	Somewhat	9 (30%)	5 (50%)	7 (36.84%)	8 (42.11%)	4 (50%)	5 (55.56%)	12 (42.86%)	7 (28%)	25 (48.08%)	
	To a large extent	21 (70%)	2 (20%)	7 (36.84%)	11 (57.89%)	4 (50%)	3 (33.33%)	9 (32.14%)	17 (68%)	21 (40.38%)	
Technical and Technological resources	Not much	0	0	2 (10.53%)	1 (5.26%)	0	0	2 (7.14%)	0	4 (7.69%)	0.2349 MC
	Somewhat	17 (56.67%)	6 (60%)	6 (31.58%)	10 (52.63%)	4 (50%)	4 (44.44%)	7 (25%)	11 (44%)	22 (42.31%)	
	To a large extent	13 (43.33%)	0	3 (15.79%)	4 (21.05%)	3 (37.5%)	3 (33.33%)	13 (46.43%)	9 (36%)	14 (26.92%)	

Challenge	Level	Col1	Col2	Col3	Col4	Col5	Col6	Col7	Col8	Col9	p-value
Legal and regulatory challenges	Not much	0	2 (20%)	2 (10.53%)	1 (5.26%)	2 (25%)	0	1 (3.57%)	3 (12%)	7 (13.46%)	0.002^M C*
	Somewhat	16 (53.33%)	0	7 (36.84%)	12 (63.16%)	4 (50%)	5 (55.56%)	19 (67.86%)	6 (24%)	25 (48.08%)	
	To a large extent	12 (40%)	4 (40%)	2 (10.53%)	0	1 (12.5%)	2 (22.22%)	2 (7.14%)	9 (36%)	7 (13.46%)	
Frequent transfer of officials	Not much	3 (10%)	0	2 (10.53%)	5 (26.32%)	3 (37.5%)	1 (11.11%)	4 (14.29%)	1 (4%)	5 (9.62%)	0.0085 MC*
	Somewhat	21 (70%)	6 (60%)	8 (42.11%)	4 (21.05%)	3 (37.5%)	6 (66.67%)	16 (57.14%)	8 (32%)	27 (51.92%)	
	To a large extent	4 (13.33%)	0	1 (5.26%)	4 (21.05%)	1 (12.5%)	0	2 (7.14%)	9 (36%)	5 (9.62%)	
Financial challenges	Not much	0	0	0	3 (15.79%)	0	0	3 (10.71%)	0	3 (5.77%)	0.0399 g^{MC}*
	Somewhat	9 (30%)	4 (40%)	5 (26.32%)	0	3 (37.5%)	3 (33.33%)	4 (14.29%)	5 (20%)	16 (30.77%)	
	To a large extent	19 (63.33%)	2 (20%)	6 (31.58%)	10 (52.63%)	4 (50%)	3 (33.33%)	13 (46.43%)	13 (52%)	15 (28.85%)	
Medical supplies	Not much	0	0	2 (10.53%)	0	0	1 (11.11%)	4 (14.29%)	0	2 (3.85%)	0.0405 MC*
	Somewhat	7 (23.33%)	4 (40%)	6 (31.58%)	5 (26.32%)	3 (37.5%)	4 (44.44%)	5 (17.86%)	10 (40%)	21 (40.38%)	

Category	Response										p-value
(demand and supply)	To a large extent	20 (66.67%)	2 (20%)	5 (26.32%)	8 (42.11%)	3 (37.5%)	3 (33.33%)	11 (39.29%)	7 (28%)	11 (21.15%)	
Inter-sectoral coordination between ministries, industry, academia, NGOs, researchers, and donors	Not much	2 (6.67%)	0	0	2 (10.53%)	1 (12.5%)	0	1 (3.57%)	2 (8%)	3 (5.77%)	0.2319 MC
	Somewhat	15 (50%)	2 (20%)	9 (47.37%)	7 (36.84%)	5 (62.5%)	6 (66.67%)	7 (25%)	6 (24%)	20 (38.46%)	
	To a large extent	10 (33.33%)	2 (20%)	2 (10.53%)	3 (15.79%)	0	1 (11.11%)	12 (42.86%)	9 (36%)	11 (21.15%)	
Political championing by Government officials	Not much	4 (13.33%)	2 (20%)	2 (10.53%)	0	1 (12.5%)	0	3 (10.71%)	1 (4%)	3 (5.77%)	
	Somewhat	13 (43.33%)	0	5 (26.32%)	7 (36.84%)	0	6 (66.67%)	8 (28.57%)	8 (32%)	20 (38.46%)	**0.0395** MC*
	To a large extent	8 (26.67%)	2 (20%)	4 (21.05%)	5 (26.32%)	5 (62.5%)	0	11 (39.29%)	9 (36%)	11 (21.15%)	
Key stakeholders	Not much	5 (16.67%)	2 (20%)	1 (5.26%)	2 (10.53%)	0	2 (22.22%)	1 (3.57%)	2 (8%)	3 (5.77%)	**0.0275** MC*
	Somewhat	12 (40%)	2 (20%)	7 (36.84%)	8 (42.11%)	2 (25%)	2 (22.22%)	19 (67.86%)	6 (24%)	21 (40.38%)	

	To a large extent	7 (23.33%)	0	1 (5.26%)	2 (10.53%)	4 (50%)	2 (22.22%)	2 (7.14%)	8 (32%)	8 (15.38%)	
Communication and dissemination of information	Not much	1 (3.33%)	0	5 (26.32%)	2 (10.53%)	2 (25%)	1 (11.11%)	3 (10.71%)	6 (24%)	3 (5.77%)	**0.0335** MC*
	Somewhat	10 (33.33%)	8 (80%)	8 (42.11%)	7 (36.84%)	3 (37.5%)	4 (44.44%)	11 (39.29%)	5 (20%)	29 (55.77%)	
	To a large extent	19 (63.33%)	2 (20%)	6 (31.58%)	10 (52.63%)	3 (37.5%)	4 (44.44%)	14 (50%)	14 (56%)	20 (38.46%)	

*Abbreviation: MC – Chi-square test with Monte Carlo simulation, * indicates statistical significance.*

From the Chi-square test, we observe that opinion about the extent of influence of Human Resources shortage, Legal and regulatory challenges, Frequent transfer of officials, Financial challenges, Medical supplies (demand and supply), Political championing by Government officials, Key stakeholders and, Communication and dissemination of information in the implementation of the NHP-2017, has a significant association with the designation.

A higher number of participants (38-56 percent) believe that all the issues including: communication and dissemination, human resources shortfall, technical/technological resources, legal and regulatory reform, frequent transfer of officials, financial challenges, medical supplies, inter-sectoral coordination between ministries, industry, academia, NGOs, researchers and donors, political championing by government officials and key stakeholders were addressed to some extent by the National Health Policy-2017 (Table 18 and Figure 28).

Table 18: The extent of National Health Policy-2017 addressing different issues

	Addressed it fully	Not at all	Somewhat
Communication and dissemination	45 (22.5%)	43 (21.5%)	112 (56%)
Human resources shortfall	44 (22%)	26 (13%)	118 (59%)
Technical/technological resources	30 (15%)	17 (8.5%)	112 (56%)
Legal and Regulatory reform	33 (16.5%)	24 (12%)	92 (46%)
Frequent Transfer of officials	19 (9.5%)	47 (23.5%)	82 (41%)
Financial Challenges	35 (17.5%)	26 (13%)	86 (43%)
Medical supplies (demand and supply)	40 (20%)	16 (8%)	88 (44%)
Inter-sectoral coordination between ministries, industry, academia, NGOs, researchers, and donors	21 (10.5%)	14 (7%)	101 (50.5%)
Political championing by Government officials	20 (10%)	40 (20%)	76 (38%)
Key stakeholders	31 (15.5%)	12 (6%)	88 (44%)

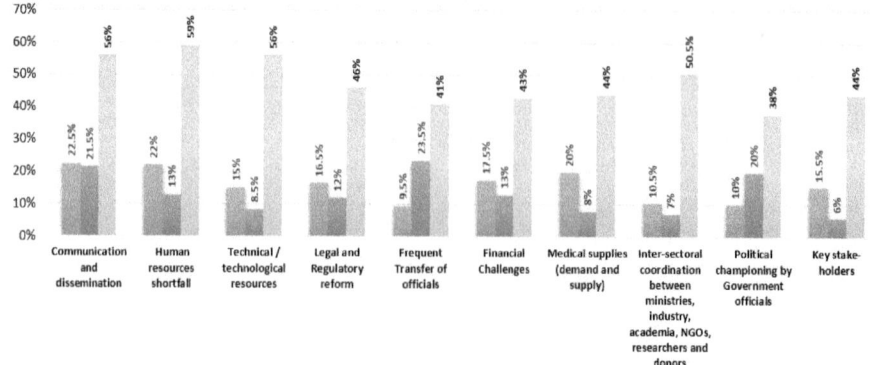

Figure 28: The extent of National Health Policy 2017 addressing different issues

The following table gives association of opinion about extent of National Health Policy 2017 addressing different issues with total experience.

Table 18 (a) : Association of opinion about extent of National Health Policy 2017 addressing different issues with total experience.

Variables	Subcategory	Between 15 - 20 years	Between 5 and 10 years	less than 5 years	More than 10 but less than 15 years	More than 20 years	p-value
Communication and Dissemination	Addressed it fully	4 (28.57%)	11 (44%)	24 (19.35%)	2 (11.11%)	4 (21.05%)	0.03998^MC*
	Not at all	4 (28.57%)	8 (32%)	23 (18.55%)	5 (27.78%)	3 (15.79%)	
	Somewhat	6 (42.36%)	6 (24%)	77 (62.1%)	11 (61.11%)	12 (63.16%)	
Human Resources Shortfall	Addressed it fully	3 (21.43%)	9 (36%)	23 (18.55%)	2 (11.11%)	7 (36.84%)	0.1284^MC
	Not at all addressed	3 (21.43%)	4 (16%)	16 (12.9%)	0	3 (15.79%)	
	Somewhat addressed	8 (57.14%)	10 (40%)	80 (64.52%)	12 (66.67%)	8 (42.11%)	
Technical / Technological Resources	Addressed it fully	3 (21.43%)	6 (24%)	18 (14.52%)	2 (11.11%)	1 (5.26%)	0.039^MC*
	Not at all addressed	2 (14.29%)	1 (4%)	9 (7.26%)	0	5 (26.32%)	
	Somewhat addressed	5 (35.71%)	10 (40%)	77 (62.1%)	11 (61.11%)	9 (47.37%)	
Legal and Regulatory Reform	Addressed it fully	2 (14.29%)	5 (20%)	23 (18.55%)	2 (11.11%)	1 (5.26%)	0.0295^MC*
	Not at all addressed	2 (14.29%)	1 (4%)	11 (8.87%)	4 (22.22%)	6 (31.58%)	

	Somewhat addressed	5 (35.71%)	11 (44%)	65 (52.42%)	6 (33.33%)	5 (26.32%)	
Frequent Transfer of Officials	Addressed it fully	0	5 (20%)	12 (9.68%)	2 (11.11%)	0	0.3333[MC]
	Not at all addressed	4 (28.57%)	4 (16%)	29 (23.39%)	5 (27.78%)	5 (26.32%)	
	Somewhat addressed	5 (35.71%)	8 (32%)	57 (45.97%)	5 (27.78%)	7 (36.84%)	
	Addressed it fully	2 (14.29%)	6 (24%)	22 (17.74%)	2 (11.11%)	3 (15.79%)	
Financial Challenges	Not at all addressed	2 (14.29%)	5 (20%)	17 (13.71%)	0	2 (10.53%)	0.5797[MC]
	Somewhat addressed	4 (28.57%)	8 (32%)	59 (47.58%)	10 (55.56%)	5 (26.32%)	
	Addressed it fully	2 (14.29%)	5 (20%)	28 (22.58%)	2 (11.11%)	3 (15.79%)	
Medical Supplies (demand and supply)	Not at all addressed	2 (14.29%)	4 (16%)	10 (8.06%)	0	0	0.2894[MC]
	Somewhat addressed	3 (21.43%)	8 (32%)	60 (48.39%)	10 (55.56%)	7 (36.84%)	
Inter-sectoral Coordination between	Addressed it fully	2 (14.29%)	3 (12%)	15 (12.1%)	1 (5.56%)	0	0.3118[MC]
	Not at all addressed	2 (14.29%)	0	11 (8.87%)	0	1 (5.26%)	

ministries, industry, academia, NGOs, researchers, and donors	Somewhat addressed	3 (21.43%)	11 (44%)	71 (57.26%)	9 (50%)	7 (36.84%)	
Political Championing by Government officials	Addressed it fully	2 (14.29%)	1 (4%)	14 (11.29%)	2 (11.11%)	1 (5.26%)	0.2049^{MC}
	Not at all addressed	2 (14.29%)	9 (36%)	23 (18.55%)	3 (16.67%)	3 (15.79%)	
	Somewhat addressed	3 (21.43%)	4 (16%)	55 (44.35%)	8 (44.44%)	6 (31.58%)	
Key Stakeholders	Addressed it fully	2 (14.29%)	2 (8%)	22 (17.74%)	2 (11.11%)	3 (15.79%)	0.0115^{MC}*
	Not at all addressed	2 (14.29%)	0	6 (4.84%)	1 (5.56%)	3 (15.79%)	
	Somewhat addressed	0	11 (44%)	64 (51.61%)	9 (50%)	4 (21.05%)	

Abbreviation: MC – Chi-square test with Monte Carlo simulation, * indicates statistical significance.

From the Chi-square test, we observe that opinion about the extent of the National Health Policy-2017 addressing Communication and Dissemination, Technical / Technological resources, Legal and Regulatory reform, and Key stake-holders related issues, have a significant association with the total experience.

The following table gives the association of opinions about the extent of National Health Policy-2017 addressing different issues with designation.

Table 18 (b): Association of opinion about extent of National Health Policy 2017 addressing different issues with designation.

Variables	Subcategory	Academician + Researcher	Civil Society Organization /NGO	Clinician	District level	National level	Private Sector	Semi-urban/ rural area	State level	Others	p-value
Communication and Dissemination	Addressed it fully	5 (16.67%)	0	4 (21.05%)	3 (15.79%)	2 (25%)	2 (22.22%)	8 (28.57%)	12 (48%)	9 (17.31%)	**0.007**^{MC}*
	Not at all	4 (13.33%)	2 (20%)	4 (21.05%)	5 (26.32%)	4 (50%)	0	11 (39.29%)	4 (16%)	9 (17.31%)	
	Somewhat	21 (70%)	8 (80%)	11 (57.89%)	11 (57.89%)	2 (25%)	7 (77.78%)	9 (32.14%)	9 (36%)	34 (65.38%)	
Human Resources Shortfall	Addressed it fully	5 (16.67%)	2 (20%)	4 (21.05%)	4 (21.05%)	0	0	11 (39.29%)	9 (36%)	9 (17.31%)	0.072^{MC}
	Not at all addressed	1 (3.33%)	0	2 (10.53%)	6 (31.58%)	2 (25%)	1 (11.11%)	5 (17.86%)	2 (8%)	7 (13.46%)	
	Somewhat addressed	24 (80%)	4 (40%)	10 (52.63%)	9 (47.37%)	5 (62.5%)	7 (77.78%)	12 (42.86%)	14 (56%)	33 (63.46%)	
	Addressed it fully	2 (6.67%)	0	6 (31.58%)	4 (21.05%)	1 (12.5%)	0	7 (25%)	6 (24%)	4 (7.69%)	**0.0205**^{MC}*

Technical / Technological Resources	Not at all addressed	3 (10%)	0	0	4 (21.05%)	0	0	3 (10.71%)	1 (4%)	6 (11.54%)	0.1279^{MC}
	Somewhat addressed	25 (83.33%)	5 (50%)	6 (31.58%)	7 (36.84%)	5 (62.5%)	7 (77.78%)	12 (42.86%)	13 (52%)	32 (61.54%)	
	Addressed it fully	1 (3.33%)	2 (20%)	3 (15.79%)	1 (5.26%)	1 (12.5%)	(0%)	7 (25%)	6 (24%)	12 (23.08%)	
Legal and Regulatory Reform	Not at all addressed	5 (16.67%)	2 (20%)	1 (5.26%)	4 (21.05%)	1 (12.5%)	1 (11.11%)	1 (3.57%)	4 (16%)	5 (9.62%)	
	Somewhat addressed	23 (76.67%)	1 (10%)	7 (36.84%)	10 (52.63%)	4 (50%)	5 (55.56%)	12 (42.86%)	8 (32%)	22 (42.31%)	
	Addressed it fully	1 (3.33%)	2 (20%)	3 (15.79%)	2 (10.53%)	1 (12.5%)	0	2 (7.14%)	5 (20%)	3 (5.77%)	
Frequent Transfer of Officials	Not at all addressed	11 (36.67%)	2 (20%)	1 (5.26%)	7 (36.84%)	2 (25%)	2 (22.22%)	5 (17.86%)	3 (12%)	14 (26.92%)	0.2564^{MC}
	Somewhat addressed	16 (53.33%)	1 (10%)	7 (36.84%)	6 (31.58%)	3 (37.5%)	4 (44.44%)	13 (46.43%)	10 (40%)	22 (42.31%)	
	Addressed it fully	9 (30%)	0	5 (26.32%)	1 (5.26%)	0	0	9 (32.14%)	5 (20%)	6 (11.54%)	
Financial Challenges	Not at all addressed	4 (13.33%)	0	3 (15.79%)	5 (26.32%)	3 (37.5%)	1 (11.11%)	6 (21.43%)	1 (4%)	3 (5.77%)	**0.0035**^{MC*}

Medical Supplies (demand and supply)	Somewhat addressed	14 (46.67%)	5 (50%)	5 (26.32%)	9 (47.37%)	3 (37.5%)	5 (55.56%)	5 (17.86%)	12 (48%)	28 (53.85%)	0.0025^MC*
	Addressed it fully	7 (23.33%)	3 (30%)	4 (21.05%)	3 (15.79%)	0	1 (11.11%)	9 (32.14%)	7 (28%)	6 (11.54%)	
	Not at all addressed	1 (3.33%)	0	1 (5.26%)	7 (36.84%)	0	0	1 (3.57%)	1 (4%)	5 (9.62%)	
Inter-sectoral Coordination between ministries, industry, academia, NGOs, researchers, and donors	Somewhat addressed	19 (63.33%)	2 (20%)	6 (31.58%)	5 (26.32%)	6 (75%)	4 (44.44%)	9 (32.14%)	10 (40%)	27 (51.92%)	0.023^MC*
	Addressed it fully	1 (3.33%)	2 (20%)	3 (15.79%)	3 (15.79%)	3 (37.5%)	0	0	6 (24%)	3 (5.77%)	
	Not at all addressed	4 (13.33%)	0	0	3 (15.79%)	0	0	2 (7.14%)	2 (8%)	3 (5.77%)	
Political Championing by Government Officials	Somewhat addressed	22 (73.33%)	3 (30%)	6 (31.58%)	9 (47.37%)	2 (25%)	5 (55.56%)	15 (53.57%)	9 (36%)	30 (57.69%)	0.1744^MC
	Addressed it fully	4 (13.33%)	2 (20%)	4 (21.05%)	1 (5.26%)	0	0	2 (7.14%)	3 (12%)	4 (7.69%)	
	Not at all addressed	4 (13.33%)	2 (20%)	3 (15.79%)	6 (31.58%)	1 (12.5%)	2 (22.22%)	9 (32.14%)	2 (8%)	11 (21.15%)	

Key Stakeholders										
Somewhat addressed	19 (63.33%)	1 (10%)	4 (21.05%)	5 (26.32%)	4 (50%)	4 (44.44%)	8 (28.57%)	10 (40%)	21 (40.38%)	
Addressed it fully	5 (16.67%)	2 (20%)	4 (21.05%)	4 (21.05%)	1 (12.5%)	0	4 (14.29%)	4 (16%)	7 (13.46%)	0.7546^{MC}
Not at all addressed	1 (3.33%)	0	1 (5.26%)	3 (15.79%)	1 (12.5%)	1 (11.11%)	2 (7.14%)	1 (4%)	2 (3.85%)	
Somewhat addressed	19 (63.33%)	3 (30%)	6 (31.58%)	5 (26.32%)	3 (37.5%)	4 (44.44%)	13 (46.43%)	9 (36%)	26 (50%)	

Abbreviation: MC – Chi-square test with Monte Carlo simulation, * indicates statistical significance.

From the Chi-square test, we observe that opinion about the extent of National Health Policy 2017 addressing Communication and Dissemination, Technical / Technological Resources, Financial Challenges, Medical Supplies (demand and supply), and Inter-sectoral Coordination between ministries, industry, academia, NGOs, researchers, and donors related issues, has a significant association with designation.

Key challenges in implementation of National Health Policy 2017

Table 19 represents the rank in order of the importance of key challenges in the implementation of the NHP-2017. Lack of clarity on goals was ranked 1st by 44.5 percent of participants, human resources shortfall was ranked 2nd (37.5 percent), work overload of healthcare workers was ranked 3rd (32 percent), inadequate training of healthcare workers was ranked 4th (36 percent), lack of coordination-siloed working was ranked 5th (33.5 percent), lack of financial resources was ranked 6th (26 percent), programs disconnected from ground realities was ranked 7th (38.5 percent), bureaucratic red-tapism and delayed decision making were ranked 8th (47.5 percent) and no freedom to try innovations was ranked 9th (56.5 percent).

Table 19: The rank in order of their importance of key challenges in the implementation of the National Health Policy-2017

Variables	Rank								
	1	2	3	4	5	6	7	8	9
Lack of clarity on goals	89 (44.5%)	37 (18.5%)	22 (11%)	10 (5%)	08 (4%)	12 (6%)	07 (3.5%)	02 (1%)	(6.
Human Resources shortfall	35 (17.5%)	75 (37.5%)	34 (17%)	17 (8.5%)	14 (7%)	10 (5%)	06 (3%)	08 (4%)	(0.
Work overload of healthcare workers	17 (8.5%)	31 (15.5%)	64 (32%)	37 (18.5%)	18 (9%)	13 (6.5%)	07 (3.5%)	07 (3.5%)	06
Inadequate training of healthcare workers	03 (1.5%)	09 (4.5%)	25 (12.5%)	72 (36%)	43 (21.5%)	23 (11.5%)	16 (8%)	08 (4%)	(0.
Lack of coordination - siloed working	08 (4%)	11 (5.5%)	17 (8.5%)	19 (9.5%)	67 (33.5%)	41 (20.5%)	19 (9.5%)	09 (4.5%)	(4.
Lack of financial resources	21 (10.5%)	09 (4.5%)	20 (10%)	24 (12%)	31 (15.5%)	52 (26%)	26 (13%)	07 (3.5%)	10 (
Programs disconnected from ground realities	12 (6%)	10 (5%)	11 (5.5%)	13 (6.5%)	09 (4.5%)	23 (11.5%)	77 (38.5%)	30 (15%)	1 (7.5
Bureaucratic red-tapism and delayed	10 (5%)	11 (5.5%)	02 (1%)	06 (3%)	04 (2%)	16 (8%)	24 (12%)	95 (47.5%)	3 (16

decision making									
No freedom to try innovations	05 (2.5%)	07 (3.5%)	05 (2.5%)	02 (1%)	06 (3%)	10 (5%)	18 (9%)	34 (17%)	113 (56.5%)

- Lack of clarity on goals
- Human Resources shortfall
- Work overload of healthcare workers
- Inadequate training of healthcare workers
- Lack of coordination - siloed working
- Lack of financial resources
- Programs disconnected from ground realities
- Bureaucratic red-tapism and delayed decision making
- No freedom to try innovations

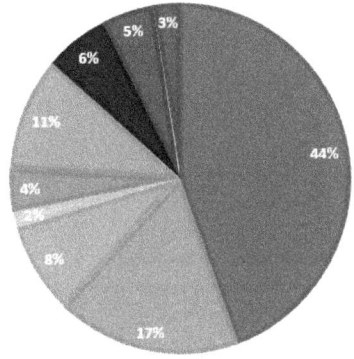

Rank* of key challenges in the implementation of the NHP-2017 (First Rank)

*(in order of the importance)

- Lack of clarity on goals
- Work overload of healthcare workers
- Lack of coordination - siloed working
- Programs disconnected from ground realities
- No freedom to try innovations
- Human Resources shortfall
- Inadequate training of healthcare workers
- Lack of financial resources
- Bureaucratic red-tapism and delayed decision making

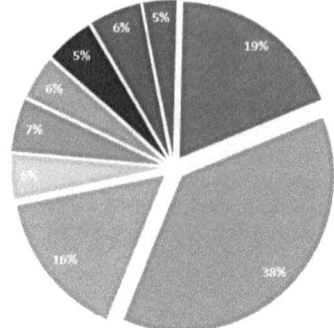

Rank* of key challenges in the implementation of the NHP-2017 (Second Rank)
*(in order of the importance)

- Lack of clarity on goals
- Work overload of healthcare workers
- Lack of coordination - siloed working
- Programs disconnected from ground realities
- No freedom to try innovations
- Human Resources shortfall
- Inadequate training of healthcare workers
- Lack of financial resources
- Bureaucratic red-tapism and delayed decision making

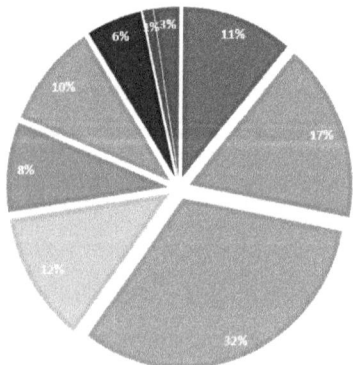

Rank* of key challenges in the implementation of the NHP-2017 (Third Rank)
*(in order of the importance)

Role of healthcare data

Table 20 and Figure 29 depict the importance of healthcare data while planning, delivering, and improving the health care sector. The majority of participants believe that healthcare data is of great importance while planning for healthcare programs (74 percent), delivering appropriate health interventions (55 percent), and improving healthcare delivery (57.5 percent).

Table 20: The role of health care data for different factors

	Planning for healthcare programs	Delivering appropriate health interventions	Improving healthcare delivery
High importance	148 (74%)	110 (55%)	115 (57.5%)
Low Importance	03 (1.5%)	01 (0.5%)	04 (2%)
Medium Importance	43 (21.5%)	46 (23%)	36 (18%)

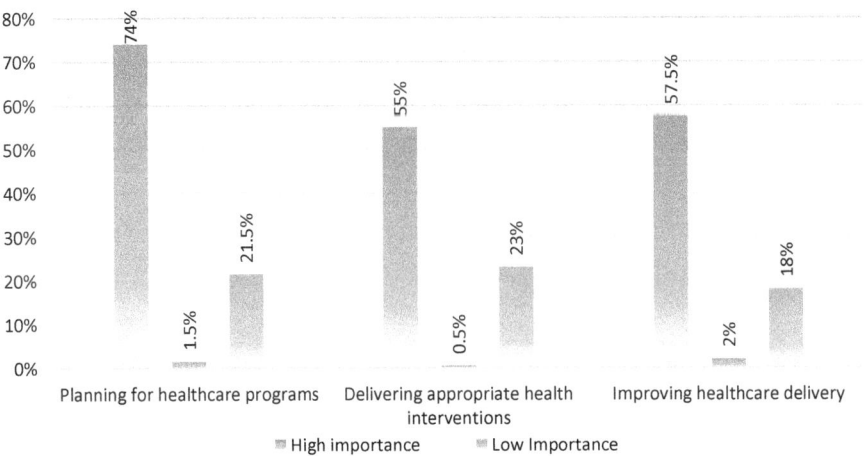

Figure 29: Role of data in planning, delivering, and improving health care

Importance of medical and paramedical professionals in healthcare delivery

Table 21 presents the importance of caregivers in health care delivery. The majority of the participants believe that Doctors, ASHA and ANMs, and nurses are of high importance in health care delivery. Pharmacists, healthcare counsellors, and AYUSH professionals are of medium importance, whereas, local unqualified practitioners/quacks are of low importance in healthcare delivery (Table 21 and Figure 30).

Table 21: Importance of medical and paramedical professionals in healthcare delivery

Care Givers	High importance	Low importance	Medium importance
ASHA and ANMs	130 (65%)	08 (4%)	55 (27.5%)
Doctors	141 (70.5%)	04 (2%)	26 (13%)
Nurses	107 (53.5%)	04 (2%)	48 (24%)
Pharmacists	72 (36%)	09 (4.5%)	77 (38.5%)
Healthcare counsellors	69 (34.5%)	11 (5.5%)	77 (38.5%)
AYUSH Professionals	52 (26%)	27 (13.5%)	78 (39%)
Local unqualified practitioners / Quacks	34 (17%)	74 (37%)	47 (23.5%)

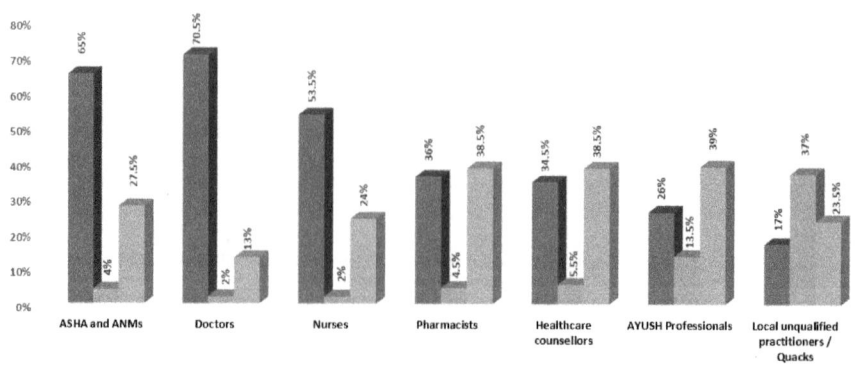

Figure 30: Importance of medical and paramedical professionals in health care delivery

Qualitative Results

Since the study is about making suggestions on Health Policy Process and its components, it was critical to seek suggestions from the study subjects which included; senior - serving and retired officials at the central, state, district, and lower levels, besides stakeholders involved in healthcare delivery. For the study subjects, qualitative inputs have been taken under the four stages of the health policy process, and captured individually from respondents across the government and private sector (without revealing their identities), to reflect their level of awareness, understanding of the policymaking process and their suggestions for its improvement.

Agenda Building & Policy Making

- Patient centricity should be the overarching theme.
- 'One Health' should become an important agenda, given the emergence of pandemics, and the zoonotic diseases.
- Cultural differences and constraints should be factored.
- Situational analysis should go beyond the desktop review, to set the agenda.
- Center-state relations should be an important consideration, and the policy should give a direction and framework for cooperation and accountability in healthcare delivery.
- Communication tools should be utilized to create awareness about the agenda-setting in the policymaking process.
- Beneficiaries should be involved in agenda-setting. The role of patient groups is important.
- Gate-keeping mechanism must be addressed.
- Problem identification should be thoroughly done, based on in-depth research on the current issues and the contributing reasons/ factors should be worked upon.
- Focus should be on marginalized and the vulnerable citizens.
- Clinical leadership issues should be addressed.
- There should be involvement of experienced doctors in the policymaking and planning.

- Make policymaking more inclusive and transparent. We must open our eyes to the real issues of quality care, reach, and affordability.
- The prerequisite to improving the policy development stage is in the recognition of the fact that policy development is a starting point for the drafting of the law. Hence, the procedures and practices for the development of policies are essential.
- Opinions from the PHCs should be considered while making policies.
- All systems of medicine should be given importance.
- Quality primary health facilities should be accessible to the rural population.
- Lack of adequate human resources, brain drain to the west, poor public healthcare infrastructure, more clinicians working for public health, emergency response, and readiness are key factors to be addressed in the NHP.
- Budget allocation and financial resources should be factored.
- There is a need for a constitution of technical groups and priority stakeholders, and this should be consulted regularly. There should be a committee formed for recommending the same. This should be vetted by a high-level committee comprising bureaucrats, public health professionals, WHO/UN representatives, researchers, etc.
- The dependency on the private health sector should be recalibrated and balanced across sectors. The planning for fund allocation should be done in terms of communicable diseases like COVID 19.
- Supply chains should be addressed to reduce import dependence on APIs and MedTech.
- 'Make in India' for manufacturing high-end devices can help address the issue of access and affordability.
- Hard and soft infrastructure gaps like lack of 24x7 power supply, should be factored.

Planning

- Planning should be short-term, and medium term factoring the long-term needs for health.
- Sectoral, domestic and global developments should be factored in planning.
- Bureau of Planning (BOP) should be revived at the MoHFW.
- Goal-based planning should be backed with proper vision.
- The policy planning process should start from grassroots levels.

- Research should be prioritized, and simplification of research approvals without compromising the ethical issues should be addressed.
- Since India is a vast country with so much diversity across the states, it is suggested to have equal representation of all states during the planning process.
- Professionals to be included in planning and follow up.
- It might be helpful to involve some medical technology representation to ensure that the emerging technologies are factored in.
- De-silo the planning process: Involvement of bodies like Telecom Engineering Centre, Bureau of Indian Standards, and NABH will be helpful to ensure that healthcare is standardized.
- More participation from the private sector, and the (pharma and med-tech) may add another perspective, since the majority of the healthcare is now being delivered by the private sector.
- The policy-making process should be made more transparent and inclusive. There should be extensive public consultations and ground level studies before finalizing the policy document.
- Not much data is available on evidence-based policymaking (as stated by a Member of Parliament and former Union Minister). This should be addressed in a planned and institutionalised manner.
- Policy goals should be developed by wider participation of think tanks, health organizations, donors etc., and by implementors.

Implementation

- Stewardship is required, both at an institutional and individual level, for the successful implementation of the health policies.
- There is an urgent need to strengthen the infrastructure & manpower.
- Career progression plan and a Succession planning must be in place to avoid vacancies.
- Strengthening of intersectoral coordination is needed.
- Improvement in the training of healthcare workers is required.
- Utilisation of equipment in public health facilities is a huge challenge.
- The need to reduce downtime of equipment with proper service by biomedical engineers is important.

- Additional charge should not be given to joint secretaries as it negatively impacts implementation.
- Digital Health tools must be deployed extensively.
- Knowledge sharing – dissemination platform should be used to share the best-practices and learning.

Monitoring and Evaluation

- Ground level awareness is needed about the Monitoring and Evaluation of Health Policies.
- Indicators should be set at the district level.
- Professionals should be included in the follow-up.
- Inter-ministerial reviewing process should be introduced.
- Audit and improvement of financial flaws should be incorporated.
- Implementation of the guidelines should be scrutinised closely, and officials related should be answerable. Health infrastructure should not be modified to accommodate the whims and fancies of politicians.
- Collection of the patient treatment data and analysis of treatment outcomes.
- Focus should be on patient engagement and shared decision making.
- Move away from siloed working and collaborate with other organizations.
- One of the key challenges in monitoring and implementation of the NHP is the distribution of responsibility for efficient monitoring and evaluation of health programs at the State level, and at the block level through community-based monitoring.
- Community monitoring and involvement of local bodies with an HMIS (Health Management Information System) is crucial for effective governance.
- Real-time dashboards should be developed. This will remove the date reporting time lag.
- Automation of the Monitoring and Evaluation process may be a good option.
- A mechanism should be put in place to fix the accountability – someone should held accountable to the public for non-implementation of the policy, or deviation from the original plan and it must be done every year.
- Intellectuals/experts with a high degree of integrity should be involved in the approval process and implementation.

- We should move away from measuring the processes to measuring outcomes. Outcome indicators should be defined and should be measured against time-bound delivery.
- Media and journalists should be considered critical to monitoring and evaluation, and citizens should be allowed to access data.
- Project Monitoring and Management Office (PMO) should be set up for M&E.
- An independent body like the CAG is needed for Monitoring and Evaluation.
- Action taken report should be filed for the findings of regular monitoring and evaluation.
- Funding to the states should be linked to the performance and improvement of health indicators.

Key Individual Inputs

Sitting Member of Parliament and former Union Minister, Government of India

- Those involved in delivering healthcare programs should not be involved in monitoring and implementation.
- MOHFW should use advanced data analytics, else monitoring and evaluation will be tough.
- Minutes of the review of the implementation plan of NHP should be shared in the public domain as this may positively impact the implementation.
- Randomly selected beneficiaries, the lowest level of health cadres, grassroots workers, CSOs (Civil Society Organizations), and independent third parties should be involved in Monitoring & Evaluation.
- Field workers have no say in monitoring and evaluation. This must be addressed.
- Review and discussion of the performance reports in the legislature should be initiated.
- Comparative assessment of districts in and across states would be helpful.
- Policy should be translated into regional languages and disseminated.

Director, MoHFW, Government of India

'I have no idea who influenced the NHP-2017. However, as per my understanding, NHP-2017 covered most of the issues and areas which can improve the health care sector in India. Also, the bureaucrats are the main implementors and planners in our country and they have a presence in international organizations as well like; WHO, World bank, etc. They drive the entire process from ideation to on-ground implementations. All the other stakeholders merely play the role of advisors, nothing else. There should be clear-cut decentralization of the process of policymaking and implementation. Politicians can play this role very well and they can drive things by utilizing the power of multiple stakeholders by authorising them to take decisions and make them accountable for the same. Authority and accountability should be given to all the stakeholders as well as implementors. In ninety percent of the cases, the officers/implementors are unable to understand what has been written in the document and what were the pertinent issues behind them, or they interpret the same as per their choice/will. Therefore, the key people/ stakeholders should be linked with the policies, and they should work as mentors/ key resource persons of the programme/ policy, till the outcome of the deliverables is achieved'.

Senior Official of MoHFW, Government of India

Health should be made a central subject: Health should become a Central Subject and necessary constitutional amendments may be made. COVID-19 is the right example to discuss the issue because, without the NDMA act, the health ministry would not have been able to perform and control the cases. So, this is the right time to make Health as a central subject.

Also, it has been observed that things are being changed at the top level due to the non-availability of funds or focus on other activities, without any consultation with actual policy planners and key resource person (s). Therefore, from day one, clear-cut availability of the funds to that division/ ministry should be provided, along with a person from the finance ministry, with all due powers to take decisions on behalf of the finance ministry.

A bigger ministry may be formed merging related ministries or all other ministries like drinking water, environment, and labour must work together with one reporting authority. Very soon, India will also be requiring a dedicated organisation with all legal backing to work for the social happiness of the citizens, including government and private employees and their work-life balance.

The Minister concerned can play the actual role of the champion. However, he needs to better understand the actual issues. It has been observed many times, that the minister is either dependent on the officers or pursuing different agendas other than related to actual issues or problems. Most of the times, officers/ ministers are not ready to fix the bottlenecks in their departments or work in ground zero.

Gram Panchayat should be on-board in monitoring and evaluation and dedicated agencies should work to monitor the programmes around the year, so that required changes or improvement can be done during the implementation of the programme phase only. Also that we need trained resources to monitor the programmes and a strong organisational setup like CAG.

There should be some independent organisation that should work with different ministries and monitor the programmes on a long term basis. Monitoring organizations should be treated as technical organisation and not a typical administrative setup. Frequent change of the head of the monitoring organisation should be avoided as it directly affects the entire process.

There is a lack of understanding of policy documents and their ownership, amongst officials.

The health ministry should plan the new policy based on long-term planning and retain the key resource person from the drafting committee. They may further be given the required powers to implement the same under their leadership.

A leading doctor and an entrepreneur in Med-Tech Space in India

'I think the public must be educated on key points of the NHP. I do not think many of my physician friends know about it in as much detail as they should'.

Senior Armed forces official from the Army Medical Corps (AMC)

'The NHP-2017 has failed to make health a justiciable right like the way it was implemented for school education through Right to Education Act 2005. So, it is time to make health a fundamental right. We need to improve the civil registration and surveillance systems which will enable us to analyse the health data from national to block level, and address major health problems based on ground level data-based inputs. Also, I am not aware of the implementation framework of the NHP-2017'.

Healthcare Leader in South & West Asia

- Co-ordination has started between the Government and the industry. However, a lot needs to be done in this respect. Cross-sectional, as well as cross-functional coordination, is the need of the hour to address the health and healthcare of the 1.3 billion population of this huge country. There must be a robust system to affect a tangible exchange between Government and the Private health care systems.
- Introduction of Technology, EHR, EMR, and Skill Development centres should be looked into.
- PPP (Private Public Partnerships) should be encouraged in all spheres of Healthcare Ecosystem - from Treatment to Manufacturing to Research, everyone needs to join hands.
- M&E Committee members are disconnected from ground realities, and this should be addressed.
- Participation of a wider population, even people outside healthcare, should be involved, to get an outside perspective.
- Patient management should be given more importance than disease management.

- Increasing the number of medical colleges and medical seats may be helpful to address the growing needs of doctors.
- Changes in medical course curriculum, and introduction of modern technology in the curriculum is imperative.
- Make in India initiative to be extended for sophisticated medical devices optimized with Indian disease patterns.
- EHR to be implemented to embark on AI and MI-based curative solutions.
- Strive to Improving the accessibility of healthcare delivery through technological interventions.

Deputy Director General – Ministry of Communication & Information Technology, Government of India

It would be better to have comments from organizations working in the domains associated with Digital Health. M2M (Machine to Machine) / IoT (Internet of Things) technology will be quite important, and these organization could give some relevant input.

ASHA workers may be trained to use the connected medical devices, through which vital parameters may be transmitted to the cloud. Data analytics and AI algorithm may be used. Problematic cases may be seen by doctors.

A complete eco-system is required to be implemented, using a National optical fibre network.

Former Additional Director General of Health Services, MoHFW, Government of India.

- Earlier policies were implemented partially.
- The number of Beneficiaries of various health programs is an indicator of utilization of services. But to measure the impact, periodic community-based surveys would be required. HMIS has been useful to assess the implementation of programs.
- Participation/data sharing in the private healthcare sector is low, and thus routine data are not representative.
- Dedicated M&E trained human resources are required for data analysis and it's reporting.

- Indicators to measure the satisfaction of beneficiaries are inadequate and cannot be measured through routine reporting. There is a need to measure these independently and give opinions to program managers and planners in a true and transparent manner
- There is a need to earmark funds for M&E of NHM and various NHPs.
- Electronic Public-Reporting Systems need to be developed for timely response to grievances.
- Periodic independent evaluation of NHP should happen at least every 5 years.
- Forum to share successful and effective innovative approaches should be developed.
- Assessment of quality of healthcare, including beneficiaries as well as non-seekers of Government healthcare services, should be done.
- More involvement of NGOs and the Private Sector is needed.
- Effective multisectoral coordination should be focused upon.
- Convergence of various National Health Programs should be done.
- We should go to the people directly and get truly anonymized online surveys. The survey should involve every stakeholder and beneficiary.
- Transparency should be brought at all levels.

Serving senior official of the MoHFW, Government of India

- Inter-sectoral coordination (between ministries, private-public partnerships, donor agencies, academics, researchers, etc.) existed before NHP-2017. However, the mechanism has been strengthened with more careful coordination with donor agencies, whose actions in some areas proved to be against national interest.
- Inter-ministerial Committees have been formed.
- Intra-ministerial committees have been formed.
- Inter-State Councils are functioning very well and with Hon'ble Home Minister being Chair of these Councils, very effective resolution of issues is happening.

Issues Needing Address:

- Alcohol, Tobacco, and e-Cigarettes ban needed all over India
- Committees headed by Additional Secretary level officers for different ministries/departments related to Health – to be formed for Joint Directives. As of now,

similar tasks are being done by different departments leading to the duplication of efforts and the wastage of resources
- PPP needs to be implemented with absolute caution and checks and balances.

Serving senior official of MoHFW, Government of India

Beneficiaries and social organizations have been observed to be minor players in the entire exercise of the policymaking process.

Notification with timeline, researching on various aspects, inviting suggestions, drafting policy document, putting it in public domain (inviting comment), finalization, approval, and release of policy documents, should be followed as a process.

We must revive the Bureau of Planning (BOP) and put it back with the Directorate General of Health Services (DteGHS) - technical wing of Ministry for such exercises, with adequate resources. The selection of human resources should be through an open advertisement with those having extensive experience working at the district, state, and central levels. Presently, after the launch of National Health Mission, this work is being done by National Health Systems Resource Centre (NHSRC), and this is a wrong policy decision. NHSRC should be dissolved. DteGHS needs to be strengthened, with DGHS as Secretary of the Department of Health. Stakeholders meeting, with adequate meeting notice and presentation should be organized at various levels and different geographical areas to capture the aspirations of all regions and sections of the society.

'I haven't seen the cost-effectiveness of health interventions influencing the planning and decision-making of the NHP-2017, and the evidence for the financial sustainability of health interventions did not influence the planning and decision-making of the NHP-2017'.

Human resources (HR) are the most important resource for effective implementation. There must be an HR Cell in the Ministry. It's unfortunate that despite observing and expressing this need by various programme managers, this work has been given to an outsourced agency that doesn't have experience of working in the field. Health Sector has a very complex working atmosphere, involving a large fleet of workers from varied fields. Presently, most of the work is being handled by the contractual staff who doesn't have ownership and sincerity because of uncertainty about their future. This is adversely affecting the implementation of various activities. Monitoring and Evaluation have not been adequately addressed in the NHP-2017 and should have the component

of a mid-term review. Most of the divisions have a M&E wing, but lack the cutting edge and is in want of finances and approvals, and the same should be addressed.

Lack of communication between different ministries is still an issue. A formal mechanism may be developed, which may also include some informal meetings.

Yearly report and monthly bulletin on the achievements of the Ministry could be a method to address this issue.

There is a need to come out with Policy Perspectives from the COVID-19 experiences. At the same time, we need to dwell on how to take care of prevalent problems likely to emerge in the coming days.

Former Executive Director of the National Health Systems Resource Centre, MoHFW, Government of India

The previous health policies have been implemented partially.

The National Health Mission has taken over the funding of all national health programs, though, its structure was never reviewed, and no changes were made. 'Mission' by definition is time-bound; this mission does not have an end date!

'The policy must look at strengthening primary healthcare, and more attention should be paid to non-communicable diseases. Health as a human right, was incorporated in the draft, but was taken out from the final policy. This should be addressed. Intersectoral coordination has been addressed in policy, but lacks implementation. I don't know if anyone is monitoring its implementation. Politicians and bureaucrats are only interested in bringing out the policy. No one wants to be responsible for monitoring the policy. The accountability framework was prepared with the policy, but is buried in the files. Mechanisms must be in place to bring accountability within bureaucracy and politicians'.

Health scenario is changing rapidly, and so is the available technology to address these. We need a dynamic policy document which could be updated every two years, based on situational analysis and review.

Clear accountability for various components of policy must be included in monitoring, otherwise it remains a document in the libraries or offices.

Former Chairman of Medical Council of India

The earlier health policies have been implemented partially, and in the NHP-2017, the problems related to health were mentioned with sketchy details in the problem statement. The NHP-2017 is not backed by robust evidence. The DGHS officials and bureaucrats have adopted the cautious approach of balancing service security with appeasement and science.

In the absence of a bottom-up approach and a robust database, which were considered as least important; although all the major problems/solutions were listed, and could have resulted in immediate state ownership and implementation, it did not happen in this way. Improper prioritization/program outline/fund allocation to states, resulted in the loss of crucial time at the state level in achieving targets, which further impacted the release of already inadequate allocation.

This issue needed clear understanding in the policy statements, with enough state-specific flexibility, which was summarily absent.

It was known to MOHFW that DGHS has been systematically weakened in the decade. Without corrective action for DGHS, one cannot efficiently administer health care delivery. Skeleton of good health governance is built on the efficient administration of service delivery, which was not touched upon in the document.

The standard processes are laid down. They are time-consuming, but essential and include; desk review, problem assessment, priority statement, gap analysis, and then the setting up of realistic goals for at least 10 years, and finally giving the policy a direction for addressing these gaps and achieving these goals. It needs to follow the democratic practice of state consultation, stakeholder consultation, and WHO/regional goals examination, so that a participatory approach is adopted. In a big country like India, with health being a state subject, it should always be preceded by people's need assessment, state-wise. People were not given adequate time in the development of NHP -2017.

Since such health policy provides direction for health care delivery, it should be led by DGHS, in consultation with the state DHS, and duly supported by bureaucrats and financial experts.

People who are working for such policy planning exercises, should be involved in every committee with their voices being heard and taken care of adequately, even at the CCH (Central Council of Health) level.

NHP-2017 was also largely aligned to the manifesto, but failed to create a synergy within the delivery of healthcare services.

The evidence with regards to the cost-effectiveness of health interventions was not factored in and did not influence the planning and decision-making of the National Health Policy 2017. Since India does not have a fully operational HTA (Health Technology Assessment) system despite the commitment in the 12th FYP, the efficacy/cost-effectiveness studies done by unscientific processes, will never justify the best use of money.

Although it is a fact that donor agencies contribute hardly 1-2 percent to the overall health budget, their influence is around 50 percent in policymaking, because they always invest in India, keeping in mind that it has a huge health products market. If we look at the charter of these donor agencies and their country of origin, it will be clear from the sub-sector, where they are investing, that all are intending to match the exporting capacity of health goods in their country. Their investment is therefore targeting to mould Indian policy for their benefit, but not for the needs of the people of India. A good trade is based on showcasing what looks like public health technology, but always securing their business profit as a priority. So, with little investment, these donor agencies influence the policy-making and secure their interests.

They work for it for years by creating infrastructure, organization, Technical Support Unit (TSU), consultants, NGO project, and data; all aimed at influencing the policy direction which suits the business interest of the country of origin of the donor organization. In absence of a robust database and HTA system, India becomes easy prey, and donor agencies become the intelligent operator.

Vaccine policy was largely based on a global direction-WHO strategy. The new vaccine integration in UIP (Universal Immunization Programme) was without immune system strengthening efforts. Research studies of adverse long-term impacts on the immune system were summarily ignored while revising the UIP.

'Similarly in other areas as well, like NCD, without robust research data – both disease burden reduction and cost reduction, happened. I am myself, a witness to not allowing the development of a national health promotion structure in India despite its approval at the Union Minister's level, which was specifically meant for disease burden and cost reduction'.

Health is a state subject, so any successful health policy should emerge from state ownership. Since it has not happened, it has adversely affected the implementation of NHP in states. Those states, which have different political party government than the centre, for those states, it is just policy rejection mindset and the states, which have the same political party government as the centre, were slow in consolidating their public health system to respond to challenges- which has left many issues unaddressed.

The beneficiaries are the first stakeholder, and their interest was addressed up to 25 percent by the NHP-2017. For the rest of the stakeholders, who get non-health dividends of any /every type, their interests were addressed 75 percent. This is happening during implementation in absence of having a structure for implementation of NHP-2017.

We must develop the following:

Functional Integrated Health Information Platform, penetrating up to village level.

Action plan for reduction of import dependence.

Technology integration in health delivery.

Build a robust public health cadre in DGHS to implement NHP.

Delegate full administrative/financial power by decentralizing it.

Director – MoHFW, Government of India

There is a scope for innovation and improvement. Technical competency must be developed at the state level for M&E. It is essentially required that stakeholders use the common M&E platform.

More community participation and convergence of other sectoral resources (IT, Media, HRD, Agriculture, etc.) are required to create and promote awareness about people's right to good health.

Director, MoHFW, Government of India

'Bureaucrats don't gel well with technocrats and Subject Matter Experts (SMEs), and this needs to be addressed. I think there is too much dependence on funding from CSR (Corporate Social Responsibility), which is not the right thing – this is just not a sustainable and scalable model. Moreover, due to the opaque nature of working at the ministry level and no accountabilities around timely decision making at this level, any such interventions can't really be sustainable.

I think that the government's aggressive price capping and profit capping measures are detrimental to the industry and will, in the longer run, harm our country by killing the introduction of new technologies and innovative solutions. A healthy demand-supply equation in a free-market setup is very much needed to drive things forward.

The policy lacks an execution blueprint and doesn't address these challenges at all'.

Private Sector Technical Expert.

One point is evident - Health needs to be the Fundamental Right of all citizens. A Policy Document must be supported with a comprehensive and granular implementation strategy, framework, and a phased implementation plan. A supportive Legal & Regulatory Framework should be developed concurrently or immediately after formulating the Policy.

Comprehensive and granular - compliance, monitoring & evaluation framework, needs to be developed and an independent agency should be created for the same.

Witnessing the current scenario of COVID-19, the challenges and impact that India is facing highlights the importance of strengthening the health management ecosystem comprehensively and building indigenous infrastructure & ecosystem to support all our national needs in health emergencies

Director-General of an independent institution of the Government of India

The implementation framework document for the policy should be a "Live" document and it should be possible to correct it mid-course.

Although the policy document at a high level has captured most details, the policy document may be updated with changing technology and availability of new devices and support to 3D print body parts. Also, home care needs to be looked at.

Director of a National Program – MoHFW, Government of India

'Probably, there is a wrong belief in the minds of all the key stakeholders for Health in India that it is the sole responsibility of the Government (both at the Centre and the states) to provide Health Services and assured Health care.

The minutes of review meetings are not shared in the public domain or discussed in public consultations and are tightly held secure by MoHFW, and hence, it seems to be not public driven. I find no mention of mid-course correction in this Policy'.

Managing Director of a leading Indian Pharmaceutical Company

'Though the objectives were right the process was incorrect. Policymaking should have relied 90 percent on doctors, patient groups, and industry experts only. Too much influence of activists and bureaucrats did a disservice to the objective. Instead of patient centricity, the policy got locked up in idealistic activists' thinking. That made pricing more important than access and destroyed the bright spot industry for the purpose of making the activist lobby happy.

If only access and patient-centricity would have been the focus, the policy implementation would have been helpful in the current dire circumstances.

Inefficiency in the system is not being tackled, as also the quality of infrastructure. Also, industry bashing is creating a bad atmosphere for investments and more dependence on China.

Please allow independent professionals for monitoring and implementing the health programs and ensure zero participation of bureaucracy in the monitoring and evaluation'.

Chairman & Managing Director of a PSU- handling Technology Implementation

New technologies like AI, AR/ VR, and Big Data Analytics could play a big role in bridging the gaps in the implementation of health programs. This applies more to the Universal Access to Health Services across Rural India.

Legal and Regulatory frameworks are important in building the confidence of both, the patients and the healthcare providers. These frameworks should have included Telemedicine as well, lack of which resulted in challenges to the healthcare professionals getting penalized and not taking it to the desired scale, resulting in widening of the gap in the services between Rural and Urban India.

1. A proper Implementation Framework formulation should become an integral part of such a policy document in future.
2. Introduce a PMO (Project Management Office) for effective Implementation monitoring and evaluation, and keep a provision for a dynamic course correction, in case it is needed.
3. The policy should be made village centric, if not citizen-centric, for a country with a rural-based setup.
4. Elaboration on leveraging the modern technologies like AI, AR/VR, 3D Printing, and e-Networks for mitigating the health-related challenges in the country, need to be emphasized.
5. Clear strategy on encouraging 'Make in India', 'Make for the World', needs to be elaborated upon.
6. More focus on policy addressing the shortage of health professionals in the country.
7. Making Telemedicine an integral part of Health domain, particularly in PPP mode, to make it more efficient and effective, with proper policy guidelines, and a legal framework to protect the interests of both, the patients and the medical fraternity.
8. District level planning is needed.
9. Professional standards for paramedics and other clinicians should be framed.
10. Vacancies should be filled on time.

Discussion

The policymaking process pertains to the initiation, specifying of policies and their organization, communication, implementation, and evaluation. Policy changes nevertheless require pragmatic adjustment of the regulations for generating new approaches to programs, with stringent measures and a provision of an altering criteria. These changes involve a complicated process, as the policymakers need to consider a variety of factors that affect their decision-making, including evidence of its impact on health, priorities of the stakeholders, feasibility, political and social considerations, and their impact on the process, and advocacy group's efforts. Utilizing an evidence-based approach to make policy decisions is significant in this complicated policy process (Tabak et al. 2015). Therefore, the objectives of this research are to study the processes involved in making a health policy and to study the involvement of various health care professionals and other stakeholders in policymaking at every level in the healthcare system.

Evidence-based studies have a crucial role in the decision-making process, while formulating the policy (Tabak et al. 2015). To date, numerous online surveys have been carried out to obtain the opinions of healthcare professionals concerning various healthcare aspects (Emanuel EJ, Emanuel LL, 1996). Therefore, the face-to-face, in-depth interviews, video conference, and online interview/survey was conducted between 2020 and 2022, with 200 participants from the health care sector. These including doctors, MBBS students, health care policymakers, laboratory technicians, journalists, and others in the health care sector. Participants with different years of work experience were included. A higher number of participants had less than five years of experience (62 percent).

Fewer number of participants with more work experiences can be attributed to their busier schedules or lack of willingness to give their input in such surveys. A higher number of participants wanted to keep their details confidential (45.5 percent) which can be directly attributed to the participants with less than five years of experience, as they fear adverse actions from superiors for sharing the factual inputs. Participants in the study represent stakeholders right from the national level to state and district and sub-district levels. Private, public, and non-government sectors were considered, spread across the states, and were selected based on their population and healthcare delivery as per the NITI Aayog's state health index. This gives a broad and deep view of the people who are important players in implementing the programs framed because of the health policies.

It is stated in the NHP-2017 that periodic surveys will be carried out to monitor the effects of policy (National Health Policy 2017). Lack of awareness and willingness to know about the policy is reflected in this study as a higher number of participants had just heard about the NHP-2017 and had not read it (42.5 percent). Moreover, despite 36.5 percent of participants having read the NHP-2017, only 12 percent of the participants had given their inputs in the surveys conducted by NHP. This also reflects negligence by the senior officials from healthcare administration, and calls for a systemic change to increase the outreach and awareness of the policymaking process. Additionally, 45 percent of the participants believed that earlier health policies were partially implemented, which might also be a reason for the participant's negligence, as a result of a lack of trust in the effectiveness of such policy documents. So, the challenge for policy planners and policymakers is to keep sharing the progress on the national health policy so that people have trust in the implementation of what is written in the national health policy.

Lack of awareness was predominantly seen in a higher number of participants (37.5 percent), and they were not aware of the healthcare problems of their area, district, or state. A shocking revelation was that, 39 percent of participants were not aware of the basis of NHP-2017 and said they would not be able to comment on it. Also, 28.5 percent of participants believed that people working at the district level and below were consulted for input. However, this sheds light on the necessity of creating awareness about the healthcare policy and building the policy with a bottom-up approach and seeking regular inputs on the implementation and impact of the provisions of the national health policy.

Along with low expenditure on health care, there are other factors such as epidemiology, policy structure, and political challenges that hinder the universal health care goal. India is burdened by both communicable and non-communicable diseases, but a sharp shift toward NCDs is reported. This change in disease pattern has implications for the health care services required because there is a need for continuous interaction with the care providers (Chakravorty et al., 2020). In the study, the majority of the participants reported that NHP-2017 addressed the issue of both communicable diseases and non-communicable diseases. A higher number of participants reported that NHP-2017 addressed primary care (49.75 percent) and planning and programming (47.72 percent). However, the participants felt that needs of tribals, backward classes, and people from hilly areas were not addressed. Rare diseases and the health of senior citizens were other areas of health that were believed to have been ignored in the NHP-2017. Quality and accessible health care include the availability of an adequate number of qualified and well-trained health care workers as per need. The situation in India is like other Asian countries where there is a shortage and abnormal distribution of health care professionals. As of 2018, in India, the density of healthcare professionals like doctors, nurses, and midwives was 25.8 per 10,000 people, as opposed to the 44.5 per 10,000 threshold as per WHO Global specification as outlined in the strategy for human resources for health to achieve the health-related Sustainable Development Goals set up in 2015.

Patchy distribution or availability of health workers across the urban and rural areas, and in the public and private sectors was also reported. This shortage of medical workforce was evident across the states like Delhi, Punjab, and states in southern India. The population density in rural India is 68 percent and when it comes to the availability of clinicians, only 34 percent of doctors and 33 percent of nurses are available in the area. Also, about 20 percent of doctors and 30 percent of nurses work in the private sector (Chakravorty et al., 2020).

NHP-2017 was built on the accomplishments of NHP 2002. "Backdrop to National Health Policy 2017-Situational Analysis", reported that NHP-2017 analysed and focused on various aspects of healthcare including; the achievements made as defined in the MDGs, Achievements in population stabilisation, disease burden, social determinants of health, inequities in health outcomes, concerns about quality of care, disease control programs, NRHM, urban health, healthcare finance, the role of non-government organizations in health, the potential of AYUSH services, the regulatory role of government, human-resource development and healthcare investments, etc. (Chakravorty et al., 2020). In the present study, a higher number of participants (49.5 percent) believed that NHP-2017 did a detailed analysis of the previous health policies. NHP -2017 believed and mentioned about utilizing the paramedics effectively. NHP-2017 had talked about various training programs, certifications, and courses for paramedics (National Health Policy 2017). The knowledge of these provisions for the utilization of paramedics was reflected among the high number of participants as they believed that role of paramedics was utilized effectively (64 percent).

NHP-2017 also aimed to educate people about the AYUSH services through digital tools (National Health Policy 2017), but a higher number of participants (44 percent) felt that AYUSH service professionals were not effectively utilized. Additionally, 81 percent of the participants felt that a separate cadre of administrative services is needed for healthcare. Therefore, this can be considered as an area of improvement while formulating the next policy. Sixty-five percent of participants believed that the issues with regards to indigenous therapies/AYUSH were addressed. Only 32 percent of participants felt that the issue about the competence of medical, nursing, and allied health professionals coming out of the private institutions were addressed.

According to the estimates, a total of 5.76 million health workforce exists which includes; allopathic doctors (1.16 million), nurses/midwives (2.34 million), pharmacists (1.20 million), dentists (0.27 million), and traditional medical practitioners (AYUSH 0.79 million) (Karan, A et al., 2021). Despite the massive health workforce, the active health workforce is much lower at 3.12 million. According to the National Health Workforce Account (NHWA), the density of doctors and nurses/midwives was estimated at 8.8 and 17.7 respectively, per 10,000 population. The density of active doctors and nurses/midwives was estimated to be 6.1 and 10.6 respectively. These numbers further dropped to 5.0 and 6.0, respectively, after filtering them for qualifications (Understanding Healthcare Access in India. 2012). Therefore, it is the need of the hour for India to invest on human resources in the health care sector to increase the active healthcare workforce and improve their quality and skillsets. This highlights the importance of investing in quality education from a policy standpoint. The country needs to encourage qualified medical professionals to join the workforce while providing opportunities for training and skill development to inadequately qualified healthcare staff.

A high number of participants (77 percent) believed that M&E is of great importance for policymaking and challenges in monitoring and evaluation includes; lack of timely and accurate data, lack of technology-driven systems, procedures, and approvals needed to share information, and too much workload. The monitoring and evaluation of health policies are important in identifying the shortcomings in health care setup and the demands of the evolving needs of the nation. This will help in designing and formulating well-informed and wholesome policies in the future. India provides a wide spectrum of quality health services, from globally renowned hospitals to hospitals that deliver uniformly poor-quality services (Krishna A, Ananthpur K., 2013).

The dearth of reliable data and technical problems in assessing quality is particularly challenging to the efforts to enhance the quality of healthcare services. Continuous efforts across the public and the private sectors aims at improving data quality, developing improved measurements and knowledge of care quality, and developing creative solutions to long-standing issues (Sarbadhikari SN. 2019). However, when the participants were asked about the quality of healthcare data in India, a majority (61.5 percent) believed that the quality of data available is average. This shows that a mission mode approach is needed to address the issues around the quality and timeliness of data. The importance of timely and quality data assumes importance, as if the data is analysed timely, interventions may be appropriate and timely and can lead to saving lives or preventing the aggravation of the disease.

A policy is only good when it is translated to ground-level implementation. As one peruses the NHP document, the last section mentions the establishment of an implementation framework to implement the commitments. A policy implementation framework would have a milestone-based roadmap with specific deliverables achieving the aims of the policy (Ministry of Health & Family Welfare, Government of India, 2017). In the current study, 52.5 percent of the participants reported being unaware of NHP-2017 having an implementation framework. Furthermore, only 54.5 percent of participants believed that NHP-2017 made a difference in healthcare. This leaves an important action point for policymakers to constantly update on the improvement of health metrics of the nations through summary updates on an annual basis.

Around 41 percent opined that NHP-2017 should be drafted for 5 years. The majority of the participants (67.5 percent) felt that every state should have its health policy. However, this agrees with the previous study conducted where it is stated that with demographical changes and shifts in disease epidemiology, the health policy has the onus for a massive reform on an urgent basis, and in a country like India, evidence-based policymaking should be considered at various levels- national, states and districts. Health should be a 'concurrent subject; give powers to the centre and the state governments to make laws' was stated by 55.5 percent of participants.

The policy articulates the establishment of organizations with adequate representation from relevant non-health ministries to reflect and institutionalize inter-sectoral coordination at all levels (the national and sub-national levels), so as to optimize the resources and maximise health outcomes. This is in line with the thinking in the emerging international "Health in All" concept, which complements 'Health for All'.
The policy mentioned empowering public health care to effectively address the factors under 'socioeconomic determinants of health' by implementing laws. Participants ranked activists (31

percent) at number one at representing the right issues in the NHP-2017, followed by NGOs/civil society organizations/charities (29 percent) at 2, World Health Organization (18.5 percent) at 3, Sustainable Development Goals (16 percent) at 4, politicians (17 percent) at 5 and patient groups (24 percent) at 6. According to the participants, state officials and paramedics, and allied health professionals had the least influence in representing the right issues in the NHP-2017.

People do believe that planning and decision-making and implementation of policy is usually influenced by various factors. This is reflected in this study as the majority of participants opined that all different factors, including; election manifesto, financial sustainability, donor funding, India's commitment to SDGs, availability of technology, new legislation, private-public partnerships, inter-sectoral coordination between ministries, private sector, academia, researchers, donors, and evidence suggesting a reduction of disease burden due to certain health interventions, somewhat influence the planning and decision making of the NHP-2017.

The majority of participants believed that human resources shortage, financial challenges, medical supplies (demand and supply), and communication and dissemination of information (46 percent) influenced the implementation of the NHP-2017 to a large extent. Furthermore, majority of participants believed that technical and technological resources, legal and regulatory challenges, frequent transfer of officials, inter-sectoral coordination between ministries, industry, academia, NGOs, researchers, and donors, political championing by government officials and key stakeholders, all influenced the implementation of the NHP-2017 to some extent. Interestingly, a higher number of participants believe that all the issues including; communication and dissemination, human resources shortfall, technical/technological resources, legal and regulatory reform, frequent transfer of officials, financial challenges, medical supplies, inter-sectoral coordination between ministries, industry, academia, NGOs, researchers and donors, political championing by government officials and key stakeholders, were addressed to some extent in NHP-2017.

A range of contrasting landscapes is depicted in the Indian health situation. In India, it is difficult to establish health equity due to pervasive discrimination and avoidable inequities ingrained in our system. Additionally, limited resources and knowledge add to poor systemic preparation to handle the issue of inequality. Hence, health policy is essential for establishing and maintaining equitable health systems.

However, when the participants were asked to rank the key challenges faced during the implementation of NHP-2017, lack of clarity on goals was ranked 1st by 44.5 percent of participants, human resources shortfall was ranked 2nd (37.5 percent), work overload of healthcare workers was ranked 3rd (32 percent), inadequate training of healthcare workers was ranked 4th (36 percent), lack of coordination-siloed working was ranked 5th (33.5 percent), lack of financial resources was ranked 6th (26 percent), programs disconnected from ground realities was ranked 7th (38.5 percent), bureaucratic red-tapism and delayed decision making were ranked 8th (47.5 percent) and no freedom to try innovations was ranked 9th (56.5 percent). According to Kasthuri et al 2018, lack of awareness about health in the general population (for example only 1/3rd of the antenatal mothers have the desired knowledge for breastfeeding, only 11.3 percent of the adolescent girls had accurate knowledge of key reproductive health issues, etc.),. lack of access to health (financial, geographic, social, and system-related barriers), lack of human resources (including inadequate numbers of personnel, unavailability of quality training, and unwillingness to serve), cost of health care, lack of accountability at every level of the healthcare community, are the major factors that are important when implementing the NHP (Kasthuri, A., 2018).

A majority of participants believed that health care data was of great importance while planning for healthcare programs (74 percent), delivering appropriate health interventions (55 percent), and improving healthcare delivery (57.5 percent). Large amounts of data ranging from information on facility to service utilization and performance indices and data on surveillance are generated by the healthcare centres. However, this data should be studied to look at the trends and indicators of functioning to understand how the quality of health care can be improved. The application of such data to guide steps in improving health outcomes was observed during the 2020 COVID-19 situation where data on the increasing number of fever cases were reported every week, but no efforts were made to understand their correlation with COVID-19 outbreaks (Asgari-Jirhandeh, N. et al., 2021).

India has a critical shortage of HRH (Human resources in Health) with about 160 skilled health workers per 100,000 population, as of 2013. India, under the Sustainable Development Goals, planned to achieve a target of 550 physicians, nurses, and midwives per 100,000 people by the year 2030. The 1978 Alma Ata declaration paved the way for the formation of the first NHPI (1983), which was subsequently revised in 2002 and 2017, to address the healthcare challenges of the country. The National Health Policy of India laid a detailed roadmap to secure the health of a billion-plus population. To improve health care outcomes in a population, focusing on strengthening the - Availability, Accessibility, Acceptability, and Quality (AAAQ), of human resources is important. Focusing on the AAAQ of health care human resources while formulating the NHP is of supreme importance in managing the shortage of human resources in healthcare.

In the present study, most participants opined that doctor, ASHA and ANMs, and nurses were of high importance in health care delivery. Pharmacists, health care counsellors, and AYUSH professionals are of medium importance, whereas local unqualified practitioners/quacks are of low importance in healthcare delivery (Table 21 and Figure 30). In line with the present study survey opinions, Dubey et al. 2021, also observed that doctors were higher in priority over auxiliary nurses-midwives and health assistants (Dubey S., et al., 2021). AAAQ indices when investigated showed a lack of healthcare workforce across all cadres over several years. Deficiency in the health care workforce was not addressed by the present NHPI recommendations. Therefore, the health care situation should be assessed based on the AAAQ indices and a stepwise framework should be implemented to address the shortage in the workforce.

The health care sector in India is at a junction where planning and development are incredibly basic in deciding the future of the nation. This sector faces significant difficulties as evident from the changing socioeconomic status of the country, condition of the public framework, absence of financial backup, lack of human resources, and unorganized administration. The amazingly low commitment of the public sector in the health care industry remains at the focal point of this issue. While the National Health Policy attempts to address most of these difficulties, execution and implementation are crucial. This study looks at the planning process for the NHP-2017. Though the public authority understands the need to increase spending on medical services, it is imperative to ensure that it takes the right direction and speed. This is a huge task for a country like India, due to its huge population, different socioeconomic class of population in each state, and the wide income disparity.

This study shed light on the policymaking process in India, its importance in developing a transparent and inclusive mechanism, and the way forward to work with all stakeholders, and guide future policymaking. Therefore, this study can be considered while designing future policies at every level.

Strengths

1. The study captures the views of parliamentarians, bureaucrats – serving and retired, clinicians across the country, people who report about health – journalists, academicians, senior government officials in health, multi-lateral bodies, civil society organizations, students in healthcare, and field level workers in healthcare. It is wide and deep both, when it comes to capturing the ground-level realities of all stakeholders. So, the findings of this research could be considered broadly representative of all key stakeholder groups.

2. Given that the study represents large, small, best performing, and poorly performing states (and Union territories), along with north, east, west, and south representation, it can be taken as a representative sample of the nation to understand the policymaking process.

3. The study is an important initiative to understand awareness among the health care sector regarding the government's policy formulation process, and implementation, and how the policy process can be improved for the effective representation of issues regarding the health sector.

4. It brings to the front the real picture of the health care sector from the point of view of an important and integral part of the sector, that is, the health care workforce.

5. The results of this survey can help in designing campaigns on the National Health Policy to target better reach, and therefore increased participation of the workforce in future policy formulations and the policy's effective implementation.

Limitations

1. There is a possibility of a distribution bias. Among 28 states, 8 Union Territories, the participants from 17 states and Union Territories were involved in this study. Also, there could have been a discrepancy in the distribution of the participants based on their location.

2. The survey did not record the registration numbers or the official email for verification in the interests of data collection. This aligns with the usual practice for face-to-face consultation from serving government or other officials, to maintain the secrecy of the respondents. Self-reporting of status was considered. The researcher believes that a respondent would not have any reason to falsify their representations.

Recommendations

Faulty planning, without a long-term policy, can inflict long-term disaster on the healthcare system. So, the key lies in following the right policymaking process. This research was conducted to assess the processes involved in making a health policy, to assess and to study the involvement of various stakeholders in policymaking, and to make recommendations for improvement in the health policy process in India. This study was conducted between 2020 and 2021 and recruited 200 participants from the health care sector, including; doctors, MBBS students, health care policymakers, lawmaker, people serving in multi-lateral bodies, academicians, bureaucrats, laboratory technicians, journalists, healthcare workers, civil society representatives, industry and professional bodies, and other stakeholders in the health care sector, across various representative states. Participants belonged to the district, state, and national level with different levels of work experience.

The findings of the research study are as mentioned below:

1. A high number of participants had heard about the NHP-2017 but 42.5 percent didn't read it, 36.5 percent had read it and 21 percent were not aware of it.
2. 40 percent of participants were not aware that the policy was available in the public domain for inputs, while 12 percent had provided their input. 45 percent of participants responded, saying that the earlier health policies have been partially implemented.
3. 28 percent of participants opined the problems of their state have been addressed in the NHP-2017, while 10.5 percent opined that the problems of their state have not been addressed in NHP-2017.
4. 34 percent of participants felt that NHP was based on data from epidemiological studies.
5. 29 percent thought that the states were consulted for inputs with regards to the NHP-2017.
6. Out of 200 participants, >50 percent reported that NHP-2017 addressed the issues related to communicable diseases and non-communicable diseases.
7. Higher number of participants reported that NHP-2017 addressed primary care (49.75 percent) and planning and programming (47.72 percent).
8. The participants felt that needs of the tribals, backward class, and people from hilly areas were not addressed. Rare diseases and senior citizens were areas of health that were believed to have been ignored in the NHP-2017.

9. Of the total, 49.5 percent feel that NHP-2017 did a detailed analysis of the previous health policies and their impact on healthcare indicators. 64 percent opined that paramedics (nurses, pharmacists, physiotherapists, etc.) were utilized effectively.
10. 81 percent thought that we need a separate healthcare cadre (like the IAS, IPS, etc.) for healthcare. 65 percent opined that the National Health Policy 2017 addressed issues with regards to indigenous therapies/AYUSH.
11. 37 percent opined that the public sector institutions churn out professionals with much better competence in medical, nursing, and allied health professionals than those coming out of private institutions. According to 32 percent of participants, NHP-2017 addressed the issue of competence of medical, nursing, and allied health professionals, coming out of private institutions.
12. 77 percent of participants opined that monitoring and evaluation are extremely important.
13. The majority of participants opined that lack of timely and accurate data (63.5 percent), lack of technology-driven systems (53.5 percent), and procedures and approvals required to share information (46.5 percent) were the key challenges in monitoring and evaluation
14. Participants ranked activists (31 percent) at number one in influencing and representing the right issues in the NHP-2017, followed by NGOs/civil society organizations/charities (29 percent) at 2. According to the participants, state officials and paramedics, and allied health professionals had the least influence in representing the right issues in the NHP-2017.
15. A majority of participants opined that all different factors, including; election manifesto, financial sustainability, donor funding, India's commitment to SDGs, availability of technology, new legislation, private-public partnerships, inter-sectoral coordination between ministries, private sector, academia, researchers, donors, and evidence suggesting a reduction of disease burden due to certain health interventions somewhat influenced the planning and decision making of the NHP-2017.
16. The majority of participants opined that the shortage of human resources, financial challenges, medical supplies (demand and supply), and communication and dissemination of information (46 percent), influenced the implementation of the National Health Policy 2017 to a large extent.
17. Lack of clarity on goals was ranked 1st by 44.5 percent of participants, human resources shortfall was ranked 2nd (37.5 percent), work overload of healthcare workers was ranked

3rd (32 percent), as the factors concerning the key challenges in the implementation of the NHP-2017.

Following recommendations emerge based on the study:

State Health Policy

Given the diversity and complexity of issues at every state, each state must frame its specific policy.

Awareness

Dissemination of information about health policy should happen through an institutionalized mechanism, targeting every stakeholder. Technology platforms, including online media channels, should be effectively utilized.

Communication and Technology

This study clearly indicates the lack of awareness about the national health policies among the masses, and so, there is a need for continuous interaction between the planners, policymakers and the public, and of regular field level studies, for timely and relevant inputs. Technology platforms must be extensively leveraged for timely communication.

Inclusive Approach

Policy inputs must be sought with thematic areas clearly mentioned, for the relevant stakeholders to share inputs. Policymaking must follow a bottom-up approach with inputs from grassroots level workers, beneficiaries, and other appropriate stakeholders. There should be involvement of individual Subject Matter Experts (SMEs), various arms of the government, CSOs, media personnel, academia, and the private sector. This will de-silo the policymaking approach and make it robust.

Quality of Data

Data has been highlighted as another major issue in Indian healthcare. Authentic and updated data is needed for making robust health policies. Epidemiology needs to be strengthened and technology could be extensively used in addressing the issue in totality. With tools of technology available, live data and dashboards should be of immense help in Implementation, Monitoring, and Evaluation. This needs a structured and institutionalized approach with adequate and appropriate human and financial resources.

Evidence-Based Policymaking – Research

Continuous research / field-level surveys are important to get feedback, which is critical for policy formulation, implementation, monitoring, and evaluation. This requires a planned approach as a part of the policymaking process and a partnership between academia, industry, and the government. Evidence should back the policy inputs and formulation.

Capacity Building

Effective policymaking requires capacity building and continuous upskilling of healthcare workers, researchers, and academia. Capacity building is an important prerequisite for effective monitoring and evaluation. Capacity building is also required for the policy formulation process, to ensure that the various components of policymaking are handled by competent professionals.

Impact Assessment – M&E

There is a need for a regular socio-economic audit of the various aspects of health policy in implementation, and suitable amends, as needed, must be made in policy post the field level impact assessment. It is critical to share the key health metrics (with regards to the achievements) with the stakeholders at every level, so that there is a sense of belongingness and ownership in them. Also, it is important to disseminate the findings among the broader network of communities so that ground-level inputs drive the formulation of future health policies through proper engagement and participation at every level.

M&E processes should be automated, and the socioeconomic impact of policies should form the basis of any mid-term policy change.

Formalizing the Policymaking Process

It is time for the government to formalize a policymaking process covering the following:

a) Agenda building and policymaking
b) Planning
c) Implementation
d) Monitoring and Evaluation.

Also, policies and programmes should have a sunset clause. The periodicity (Timelines) of the monitoring and evaluation and policy formulation must be specified, given that the previous health policies have been at irregular intervals. In the age of technology proliferation, health policies should be 'live documents', revised - based on the impact assessment, through monitoring and evaluation, and backed by the real-world evidence.

Bibliography

Gupta, R. P. (2016). *Healthcare Reforms in India: Making up for the lost decades.* Gurgaon: Reed Elsevier India Pvt. Ltd.

World Health Organization . (2005). *Designing Health Financing Systems to Reduce Catastrophic Health Expenditure.* Geneva: WHO.

Ministry of Health & Family Welfare, Government of India. (2017). *National Health Policy 2017.* New Delhi: Ministry of Health & Family Welfare, Government of India.

Srinivasan, P. (1995). National health policy for traditional medicine in India . *World Health Forum, 16,* 190-193.

Gilson, L. (2012). Health Policy and Systems Research : a methodology reader. Geneva, Switzerland: WHO Document Production Services.

WHO. (2017, February 26). *National health policies, strategies and plans.* Retrieved February 26, 2017, from WHO International : http://www.who.int/nationalpolicies/processes/en/

Exworthy, M. (2008). Policy to tackle the social determinants of health: using conceptual models to understand the policy process. . *Health Policy and Planning, 23*(5), 318-327.

National Health Authrority. (2021). *About NHA.* Retrieved November 20, 2021, from NHA: https://pmjay.gov.in/about/nha

National Health Mission. (n.d.). *NHM - NHP 2002.* Retrieved November 20, 2021, from National Health Mission: https://nhm.gov.in/images/pdf/guidelines/nrhm-guidelines/national_nealth_policy_2002.pdf

Gupta, R. P. (2016). *Health Care Reforms in India: Making up for the Lost Decades.* New Delhi: Reed Elsevier India Pvt. Ltd.

O'Connell, T., Rasanathan, K., & Chopra, M. (2014, January 18). What does universal health coverage mean? *Lancet,* 277-9. doi:10.1016/S0140-6736(13)60955-1

Azline, A., Abdullah, K. A., Iszaid, I., & Syahira, S. (2018, June). Policy Arena of Health Policy-Making in Developing Countries. *International Journal of Public Health and Clinical Sciences.*

Ministry of Health and Family Welfare, Government of India. (2021, February 12). *Ministry of Health and Family Welfare, Government of India.* Retrieved from Press Information Bureau, Government of India: https://www.pib.gov.in/PressReleasePage.aspx?PRID=1697441

Ministry of Health & Family Welfare, Government of India. (2021, March 23). *PIB, Government of India.* Retrieved from Press Information Bureau: https://pib.gov.in/PressReleasePage.aspx?PRID=1706904

Ministry of Health & Family Welfare, Government of India. (2022). *National Family Health Survey -5 : 2019-21.* Mumbai: International Institute for Population Sciences.

Ministry of Statistics & Progamme Implementation, Government of India. (2021, November 29). *An Overview of the SDGs.* Retrieved from Ministry of Statistics & Progamme Implementation, Government of India.: http://mospi.nic.in/overview-sdgs

UNDP. (2021). *SDGs*. Retrieved from UNDP: https://www.undp.org/sustainable-development-goals?utm_source=EN&utm_medium=GSR&utm_content=US_UNDP_PaidSearch_Brand_English&utm_campaign=CENTRAL&c_src=CENTRAL&c_src2=GSR&gclid=CjOKCQiAkZKNBhDiARIsAPskOWj6ow8B4UVpycNAvn2qTJakLfGX8SCxq30dBRUu4BwcuF-TOViHOV

Marchal, B., Arcens, M. T., Coates, A., & Brouwere, V. D. (2005). *An institutional analysis of the safe motherhood policymaking process in Burkina Faso*. Retrieved 12 21, 2021, from https://researchgate.net/profile/vincent_debrouwere/publication/234033327_institutional_analysis_of_safe_motherhood_in_burkina_faso_an_institutional_analysis_of_the_safe_motherhood_policymaking_process_in_burkina_faso/links/09e4150e69fbebca85000000.pdf

Jain, B., Hiligsmann, M., Mathew, J. L., & Evers, S. M. (2014). Analysis of a Small Group of Stakeholders Regarding Advancing Health Technology Assessment in India. *Value in health regional issues, 3*, 167-171. Retrieved 12 21, 2021, from https://sciencedirect.com/science/article/pii/s2212109914000272

Rameshwaram, G. (1989). *Medical and Health Administration in Rural India*. New Delhi, India: Ashish Publishing House.

Harrison, M. (1994). *Public Health in British India : Anglo-Indian preventive medicine 1859-1914*. New York, NY, USA: Cambridge University Press.

Brownson, R. C., Chriqui, J. F., & Stamatakis, K. A. (2009). Understanding Evidence-Based Public Health Policy. *American Journal of Public Health, 99*(9), 1576-1583. Retrieved 12 21, 2021, from https://ncbi.nlm.nih.gov/pmc/articles/pmc2724448

National Commission on Macroeconomics and Health. (2005). *National Commission on Macroeconomics and Health*. New Delhi: Ministry of Health & Family Welfare, Government of India.

Ministry of Health & Family Welfare, Government of India. (2013). *Annual Report 2012-13*. New Delhi: Ministry of Health & Family Welfare, Government of India.

Ghosh, A. (2001). The Rise and Fall of the National Health Policy . *Indian Anthroplogist* , 27-47.

Planning Commission of India. (2011). *High Level Expert Group Report on Universal Health Coverage for India*. New Delhi: Planning Commission of India.

Weil, D. N. (2005, July). Accounting for the effect of Health on Economic Growth. *NBER Working Paper Series*. Cambridge, MA, USA: National Bureau of Economic Research .

Commission on Growth and Development. (2008). *The Growth Report*. Washington DC.: World Bank.

Walt, G., Shiffman, J., Schneider, H., Murray, S. F., Brugha, R., Gilson, L., . . . Gilson, L. (2008). Doing health policy analysis: methodological and conceptual reflections and challenges. *Health Policy and Planning, 23*(5), 308-317. Retrieved 12 21, 2021, from https://academic.oup.com/heapol/article/23/5/308/617219

Deptt. of Health & Family Welfare, MOHFW, GOI. (2014). *Annual Report 2013-14*. New Delhi: Deptt. of Health & Family Welfare, MOHFW, GOI.

Dr.D.K.Taneja. (2013). *Health Policies and Programmes in India* (Vol. 11). (B. Banerjee, Ed.) Delhi, Delhi, India: Doctors Publications (Regd.).

Deptt. of Health & Family Welfare, MOHFW, Govt. of India. (2013). *Annual Report 2013-14.* New Delhi: Deptt. of Health & Family Welfare, MOHFW, Govt. of India.

National Health Policy. (2002). *National Health Policy, 2002.* New Delhi: Department of Health, Ministry of Health & Family Welfare, Government of India.

Ministry of Health & Family Welfare, Government of India. (2017). *National Health Policy 2017.* New Delhi: Ministry of Health & Family Welfare, Government of India.

Gupta, A. S. (2002). National Health Policy 2002: A brief critique. *The National Medical Journal of India, 15*(4), 215-16.

NITI Aayog. (2019). *Healthy States . Progressive India.* New Delhi: NITI Aayog. Retrieved October 20, 2021, from http://social.niti.gov.in/uploads/sample/SHI_Round_one percent20_Report.pdf

Ministry of Health & Family Welfare, Government of India. (2019, December 11). *Health & Wellness Centres.* Retrieved August 14, 2021, from https://ab-hwc.nhp.gov.in/#about

Chhetri, D. and Zacarias, F., 2021. Advocacy for Evidence-Based Policy-Making in Public Health: Experiences and the Way Forward. Journal of Health Management, 23(1), pp.85-94.

Johnson, S.A., 2009. Public health advocacy [Discussion Paper]. Alberta Health Services.

De Leeuw, E., Clavier, C. and Breton, E., 2014. Health policy–why research it and how: health political science. Health research policy and systems, 12(1), pp.1-11.

Delhi, N., 2002. Ministry of Health and Family Welfare, Government of India; 2002. Government of India. National Health Policy.

Sabatier, P.A. and Jenkins-Smith, H.C. eds., 1993. Policy change and learning: An advocacy coalition approach. Westview press.

Azline, A., Iszaid, I., Syahira, S., Awad, H. and Juni, M.H., 2018. Policy arena of health policy-making process in developing countries. International Journal of Public Health and Clinical Sciences, 5(3), pp.32-48.

Timmermans, A., 2001. Arenas as institutional sites for policymaking: Patterns and effects in comparative perspective. Journal of Comparative Policy Analysis: Research and Practice, 3(3), pp.311-337.

Bulger RE, Meyer Bobby E, Fineberg HV, editors. (1995). The Formulation of Health Policy by the Three Branches of Government. In Institute of Medicine (US) Committee on the Social and Ethical Impacts of Developments in Biomedicine; Society's Choices: Social and Ethical Decision Making in Biomedicine. National Academies Press.

Separation of Powers. Legislative, Executive, Judicial. (2018). National Conference of State Legislatures. *Separation of Powers | Legislative, Executive, Judicial (ncsl.org)*.

Tabak, R.G., Eyler, A.A., Dodson, E.A. and Brownson, R.C., 2015. Accessing evidence to inform public health policy: a study to enhance advocacy. Public health, 129(6), pp.698-704.

Pillai, R.K., 2016. Methodology for health policy development: introductory paper. Journal of Pharmacovigilance.

Gopalan, S.S., Mohanty, S. and Das, A., 2011. Challenges and opportunities for policy decisions to address health equity in developing health systems: case study of the policy processes in the Indian state of Orissa. International Journal for Equity in Health, 10(1), pp.1-11.

Franco-Trigo, L., Fernandez-Llimos, F., Martínez-Martínez, F., Benrimoj, Sl., Sabater-Hernández, D., 2020. Stakeholder analysis in health innovation planning processes: A systematic scoping review. Health Policy, 124(10), pp.1083-1099.

Menon, G.R., Singh, L., Sharma, P., Yadav, P., Sharma, S., Kalaskar, S., et al., 2019. National Burden Estimates of healthy life lost in India, 2017: an analysis using direct mortality data and indirect disability data. Lancet Glob Health, e1675-e1684.

Maternal health. UNICEF's concerted action to increase access to quality maternal health services. Unicef. India. *Maternal health | UNICEF India*

UNICEF Data: Monitoring the situation of children and women. Unicef. *India (IND) - Demographics, Health & Infant Mortality - UNICEF DATA*

Life expectancy at birth-India, 2021. The World Bank. Data. *Life expectancy at birth, male (years) - India | Data (worldbank.org)*.

Tarun Gidwani. National Family Health Survey (NFHS-4) 2015-16: India, 2017. Ministry of Health and Family Welfare. *https://ruralindiaonline.org/en/library/resource/national-family-health-survey-nfhs-4-2015-16-india/*

Narain J. P. (2016). Public Health Challenges in India: Seizing the Opportunities. Indian journal of community medicine: official publication of Indian Association of Preventive & Social Medicine, 41(2), 85–88. https://doi.org/10.4103/0970-0218.177507

Selvaraj, S., Karan, A.K., Mao, W. et al., 2021. Did the poor gain from India's health policy interventions?

Evidence from benefit-incidence analysis, 2004–2018. Int J Equity Health 20, 159.

Duggal, R., 2001. Evolution of health policy in India. Centre for Enquiry into Health and Allied Themes.

Delhi, N., 1983. Ministry of Health and Family Welfare, Government of India; 1987. Department of Health. Act, 47.

MoHFW.2002. Delhi: Ministry of Health and Family Welfare, Government of India; 2002. National Health Policy

The National Health Bill: Ministry of Health and Family Welfare, Government of India. 2009

Pritchett, L., 2009. Is India a flailing state? detours on the four-lane highway to modernization.

Gwatkin, D.R., 2000. Health inequalities and the health of the poor: what do we know? What can we do? Bulletin of the world health organization, 78, pp.3-18.

Ayushman Bharat - Health and Wellness Centre, 2019. Ministry of Health and Family Welfare. Government of India. *https://ab-hwc.nhp.gov.in/home/aboutus*.

National Health Authority

National Health Systems Resource Centre

National Institute of Health and Family Welfare

Indian Council of Medical Research.

Institute of Applied Medical Research.

Ayushman Bharat - Health and Wellness Centre, 2019. Ministry of Health and Family Welfare. Government of India. https://ab-hwc.nhp.gov.in/home/aboutus.

Marten, R., McIntyre, D., Travassos, C., Shishkin, S., Longde, W., Reddy, S., et al., 2014. An assessment of progress towards universal health coverage in Brazil, Russia, India, China, and South Africa (BRICS). Lancet, 384, pp.2164–71

Wang, K.M., 2011. Health care expenditure and economic growth: Quantile panel-type analysis. Economic Modelling, 28(4), pp.1536-1549.

Jakovljevic, M., Camilleri, C., Rancic, N., Grima, S., Jurisevic, M., Grech, K. and Buttigieg, S.C., 2018. Cold war legacy in public and private health spending in Europe. Frontiers in public health, 6, p.215.

Golechha, M., 2015. Healthcare agenda for the Indian government. The Indian journal of medical research, 141(2), p.151.

Nair, H. and Panda, R., 2011. Quality of maternal healthcare in India: Has the National Rural Health Mission made a difference? Journal of global health, 1(1), p.79.

Mortality rate, infant (per 1,000 live births) – India, 2021. The World Bank. Data. Mortality rate, infant (per 1,000 live births) - India | Data (worldbank.org).

Natalie Carvalho and Slawa Rokicki, 2019. The Impact of India's Janani Suraksha Yojana Conditional Cash Transfer Programme: A Replication Study, The Journal of Development Studies, 55:5, 989-1006.

Srivastava, R.K. and Bachani, D., 2011. Burden of NCDs, policies and programme for prevention and control of NCDs in India. Indian journal of community medicine: official publication of Indian Association of Preventive & Social Medicine, 36(Suppl1), p.S7.

Chatterjee, P., 2014. Manifestos for health: what the Indian political parties have promised. Bmj, 348.

Girvin, B., 2020. From civic pluralism to ethnorcligious majoritarianism. Majority nationalism in India. Nationalism and Ethnic Politics, 26(1), pp.27-45.

Planning Commission, 2011. High level expert group report on universal health coverage for India (No. id: 4646).

O'Connell, T., Rasanathan, K. and Chopra, M., 2014. What does universal health coverage mean? The Lancet, 383(9913), pp.277-279.

Golechha, M., 2014. Priorities for the next Indian government's reform of healthcare. Bmj, 348.

Dandona, L., Katoch, V.M. and Dandona, R., 2011. Research to achieve health care for all in India. The Lancet, 377(9771), pp.1055-1057

Banerjee A., 2020. Equity and Quality of Health-care Access: Where Do We Stand and the Way Forward? Indian journal of community medicine: official publication of Indian Association of Preventive & Social Medicine, 45(1), 4–7.

Nandan, D. and Agarwal, D., 2012. Human resources for health in India: urgent need for reforms. Indian journal of community medicine: official publication of Indian Association of Preventive & Social Medicine, 37(4), p.205.

Rao, K.D., Bhatnagar, A. and Berman, P., 2012. So many, yet few: human resources for health in India. Human resources for health, 10(1), pp.1-9.

Golechha, M., 2015. Healthcare agenda for the Indian government. The Indian journal of medical research, 141(2), p.151.

Mudaliar Committee. 1962. Report of the Health Survey and the Planning Committee. Government of India, Ministry of Health.

Batliwala S. 1978. The historical development of health services in India. FRCH, Bombay.

Chadha Committee, 1963. Special Committee for NMEP Maintenance Phase. MoHFW, GOI, New Delhi.

Banerji, D., 1973. Population planning in India: National and foreign priorities. International Journal of Health Services, 3(4), pp.773-777

Mukherjee Committee, 1966. Committee to Review Staffing Pattern and Financial Provision under Family Planning Programme. MoHFW, New Delhi.

Singh, K., 1973. Report of the Committee on Multipurpose Workers Under the Health and Family Planning Programme. New Delhi, Government of India, Ministry of Health and Family Planning, p.21.

Shrivastava Committee, 1975: Report of the Group on Medical Education and Support Manpower, MoHFW, New Delhi

Nandraj, S. and Duggal, R., 1996. Physical standards in the private health sector. Radical Journal of Health, 2(2/3), pp.141-84.

Kannan, K.P., Thankappan, K.R., Ramankutty, V. and Aravindan, K.P., 1991. Health and development in rural Kerala. Trivandrum: Kerala Sastra Sahitya Parishad.

NCAER. 1991. Household Survey of Medical Care, National Council for Applied Economic Research, New Delhi

High Level Expert Group Report on Universal Health Coverage

for India, 2011. Planning Commission of India. *hleg_report.pdf (uhc-india.org)*

Finlay, J., 2007. The Role of Health in Economic Development. Program on the Global Demography of Aging. PGDA Working Paper No. 21, Baldacci, E.B., 2004. The impact of Poor Health on Total Factor Productivity. The Journal of Development Studies 42 (6). 918 –938.

Government expenditure on education, total (percent of GDP). The World Bank. Data. *Government expenditure on education, total (percent of GDP) - India | Data (worldbank.org)*.

Current health expenditure (percent of GDP) – India. The World Bank. Data. *Current health expenditure (percent of GDP) - India | Data (worldbank.org)*.

Mishra, P K; Mishra, S K. The Triangulation Dynamics Between Education, Health and Economic Growth in India. ***The Journal of Commerce***; Lahore *Vol. 7, Iss. 2,* (Apr 2015): 69-89

Human Development Reports, 2020. United Nations Development Programme. *| Human Development Reports (undp.org)*.

Haque S, Singh RB. Air pollution and human health in Kolkata, India: a case study. Climate. 2017;77(5):1–16.

United Nations. Department of International Economic, United Nations. Department for Economic, Social Information, Policy Analysis. World population prospects. United Nations, Department of International, Economic and Social Affairs; [Internet] 1998. Available from: *https://www.un.org/development/desa/publications/world-population-prospects-the-2017-revision.html*).

Kalita A, Shinde S, Patel V. Public health research in India in the new millennium: A bibliometric analysis. Global health action. 2015 Dec 1;8(1):27576.

Central Bureau of health Intelligence. National health profile 2016. Directorate General of Health Services, Ministry of Health and Family Welfare. [Internet] 2016 Available from *http://www.indiaenvironmentportal.org.in/files/file/National percent20Health percent20Profile percent202016212.pdf*.

Planning Commission. Report of the steering committee on health for the 12th five-year plan. Health division, Government of India. [Internet] 2012. Available from: *https://niti.gov.in/planningcommission.gov.in/docs/aboutus/committee/strgrp12/str_health0203.pdf*.

Central Bureau of health Intelligence. National health profile 2018. Directorate General of Health Services, Ministry of Health and Family Welfare. [Internet] 2018 Available from *http://www.cbhidghs.nic.in/WriteReadData/l892s/Before percent20Chapter1.pdf*.

Bajpai V. National Health Policy, 2017. Economic & Political Weekly. 2018 Jul 14;53(28):31.

Government of India. Situation analysis: backdrop to the national health policy 2017, Ministry of Health and Family welfare. [Internet] 2017. Available from *https://mohfw.gov.in/sites/default/files/71275472221489753307.pdf*

World Health Organization. World health statistics. [Internet] 2010. Available from *https://www.who.int/gho/publications/world_health_statistics/EN_WHS10_Full.pdf*.

National Health Policy, 2017. Ministry of Health and Family Welfare. Government of India. *national_health_policy_2017.pdf (nhp.gov.in)*.

Gupta, R.K. and Kumari, R., 2017. National health policy 2017: an overview. JK Science, 19(3), pp.135-136.

Planning Commission. 2012. Report of the steering committee on health for the 12th five-year plan.

Planning Commission. 2013a. Twelfth five-year plan (2012–2017) faster, more inclusive and sustainable growth, 1:1–370.

Planning Commission. 2013b Twelfth five-year plan (2012–2017) faster, more inclusive and sustainable growth, 2:1–438.

Niti Aayog.

National Rural Health Mission (NRHM), 2021. *National Rural Health Mission (NRHM) — Vikaspedia*).

National Health Mission, 2018.

National Rural Health Mission.2020 Critical Review of the Mission Implementation and Achievements.

Kulkarni P. 2014. National Urban Health Mission: An Effort to Achieve Equity in Health. Annals of Community Health.

Highlights of Economical Survey 2020- 2021. 2021.

Bhaumik S. Health and beyond strategies for a better India: incorporating evidence to strengthen health policy. J Family Med Prim Care. 2014 Oct-Dec;3(4):313-7.

De, M., Taraphdar, P., Paul, S. and Halder, A., 2016. Awareness of breast feeding among mothers attending antenatal OPD of NRS medical college. IOSR J of Dent and Med Sci, 15, pp.3-8.

Pandey, D., Sardana, P., Saxena, A., Dogra, L., Coondoo, A. and Kamath, A., 2015. Awareness and attitude towards breastfeeding among two generations of Indian women: a comparative study. PloS one, 10(5).

Mittal, K. and Goel, M.K., 2010. Knowledge regarding reproductive health among urban adolescent girls of Haryana. Indian journal of community medicine: official publication of Indian Association of Preventive & Social Medicine, 35(4), p.529.

Tamanna, M.Z., Eram, U., Al Harbi, T.M., Alrashdi, S.A., Khateeb, S.U., Aladhrai, S.A. and Hussain, A.M., 2012. Clinical value of leukocyte counts in evaluation of patients with suspected appendicitis in emergency department. Ulus Travma Acil Cerrahi Derg, 18(6), pp.474-478.

Banerjee, S.K., Andersen, K.L., Warvadekar, J. and Pearson, E., 2013. Effectiveness of a behavior change communication intervention to improve knowledge and perceptions about abortion in Bihar and Jharkhand, India. International perspectives on sexual and reproductive health, pp.142-151.

Kotwal N, Khan N, Kaul S. 2014. A review of the effectiveness of theinterventions on adolescent reproductive health in developing countries.

Oxford Dictionary Online

Gulliford, M., Figueroa-Munoz, J., Morgan, M., Hughes, D., Gibson, B., Beech, R. and Hudson, M., 2002. What does' access to health care'mean? Journal of health services research & policy, 7(3), pp.186-188.

Munjanja, S.P., Magure, T. and Kandawasvika, G., 2012. 11 Geographical Access, Transport and Referral Systems. Maternal and perinatal health in developing countries, p.139.

Understanding Healthcare Access in India. 2012. Report by the IMS Institute for Healthcare Informatics.

Krishna A, Ananthpur K. Globalization, Distance and Disease: Spatial Health Disparities in Rural India. Millennial Asia. 2013;4(1):3-25. doi:*10.1177/0976399613480879*

Rao, M., Rao, K.D., Kumar, A.S., Chatterjee, M. and Sundararaman, T., 2011. Human resources for health in India. The Lancet, 377(9765), pp.587-598.

Rao KD.2011. Situation Analysis of the Health Workforce in India. Human Resources Technical Paper I. Public Health Foundation of India. 2011

Rural health statistics 2019-2020. 2020

Balarajan, Y., Selvaraj, S. and Subramanian, S.V., 2011. Health care and equity in India. The Lancet, 377(9764), pp.505-515.

Reddy, K.S., Patel, V., Jha, P., Paul, V.K., Kumar, A.S., Dandona, L. and Lancet India Group for Universal Healthcare, 2011. Towards achievement of universal health care in India by 2020: a call to action. The Lancet, 377(9767), pp.760-768.

Tabak, R.G., Eyler, A.A., Dodson, E.A. and Brownson, R.C., 2015. Accessing evidence to inform public health policy: a study to enhance advocacy. Public health, 129(6), pp.698-704.

Emanuel EJ, Emanuel LL. What is accountability in health care? Ann Intern Med. 1996;124:229–39.

Chakravorty, I., Daga, S., Dave, S., Chakravorty, S., Menon, G., Bhala, N., Mehta, R. and Bamrah, J.S., 2020. An online survey of healthcare professionals in the COVID-19 Pandemic in the UK. Sushruta Journal of Health Policy & Opinion, 13(2).

Karan, A., Negandhi, H., Hussain, S. et al. 2021. Size, composition and distribution of health workforce in India: why, and where to invest? Hum Resour Health **19,** 39

Understanding Healthcare Access in India. 2012 Report by the IMS Institute for Healthcare Informatics. 2012.

Sarbadhikari SN. 2019. Digital health in India – As envisaged by the National Health Policy (2017).

Kasthuri, A., 2018. Challenges to healthcare in India-The five A's. Indian journal of community medicine: official publication of Indian Association of Preventive & Social Medicine, 43(3), p.141.

Asgari-Jirhandeh, N., Zapata, T. and Jhalani, M., 2021. Strengthening Primary Health Care as a Means to Achieve Universal Health Coverage: Experience from India. Journal of Health Management, 23(1), pp.20-30.

Dubey, S., Vasa, J. and Zadey, S., 2021. Do health policies address the availability, accessibility, acceptability, and quality of human resources for health? Analysis of three decades of National Health Policy of India.

Recommendations

Faulty planning, without a long-term policy, can inflict long-term disaster on the healthcare system. So, the key lies in following the right policymaking process. This research was conducted to assess the processes involved in making a health policy, to assess and to study the involvement of various stakeholders in policymaking, and to make recommendations for improvement in the health policy process in India. This study was conducted between 2020 and 2021 and recruited 200 participants from the health care sector, including; doctors, MBBS students, health care policymakers, lawmaker, people serving in multi-lateral bodies, academicians, bureaucrats, laboratory technicians, journalists, healthcare workers, civil society representatives, industry and professional bodies, and other stakeholders in the health care sector, across various representative states. Participants belonged to the district, state, and national level with different levels of work experience.

The findings of the research study are as mentioned below:

1. A high number of participants had heard about the NHP-2017 but 42.5 percent didn't read it, 36.5 percent had read it and 21 percent were not aware of it.
2. 40 percent of participants were not aware that the policy was available in the public domain for inputs, while 12 percent had provided their input. 45 percent of participants responded, saying that the earlier health policies have been partially implemented.
3. 28 percent of participants opined the problems of their state have been addressed in the NHP-2017, while 10.5 percent opined that the problems of their state have not been addressed in NHP-2017.
4. 34 percent of participants felt that NHP was based on data from epidemiological studies.
5. 29 percent thought that the states were consulted for inputs with regards to the NHP-2017.
6. Out of 200 participants, >50 percent reported that NHP-2017 addressed the issues related to communicable diseases and non-communicable diseases.
7. Higher number of participants reported that NHP-2017 addressed primary care (49.75 percent) and planning and programming (47.72 percent).
8. The participants felt that needs of the tribals, backward class, and people from hilly areas were not addressed. Rare diseases and senior citizens were areas of health that were believed to have been ignored in the NHP-2017.

9. Of the total, 49.5 percent feel that NHP-2017 did a detailed analysis of the previous health policies and their impact on healthcare indicators. 64 percent opined that paramedics (nurses, pharmacists, physiotherapists, etc.) were utilized effectively.
10. 81 percent thought that we need a separate healthcare cadre (like the IAS, IPS, etc.) for healthcare. 65 percent opined that the National Health Policy 2017 addressed issues with regards to indigenous therapies/AYUSH.
11. 37 percent opined that the public sector institutions churn out professionals with much better competence in medical, nursing, and allied health professionals than those coming out of private institutions. According to 32 percent of participants, NHP-2017 addressed the issue of competence of medical, nursing, and allied health professionals, coming out of private institutions.
12. 77 percent of participants opined that monitoring and evaluation are extremely important.
13. The majority of participants opined that lack of timely and accurate data (63.5 percent), lack of technology-driven systems (53.5 percent), and procedures and approvals required to share information (46.5 percent) were the key challenges in monitoring and evaluation
14. Participants ranked activists (31 percent) at number one in influencing and representing the right issues in the NHP-2017, followed by NGOs/civil society organizations/charities (29 percent) at 2. According to the participants, state officials and paramedics, and allied health professionals had the least influence in representing the right issues in the NHP-2017.
15. A majority of participants opined that all different factors, including; election manifesto, financial sustainability, donor funding, India's commitment to SDGs, availability of technology, new legislation, private-public partnerships, inter-sectoral coordination between ministries, private sector, academia, researchers, donors, and evidence suggesting a reduction of disease burden due to certain health interventions somewhat influenced the planning and decision making of the NHP-2017.
16. The majority of participants opined that the shortage of human resources, financial challenges, medical supplies (demand and supply), and communication and dissemination of information (46 percent), influenced the implementation of the National Health Policy 2017 to a large extent.
17. Lack of clarity on goals was ranked 1st by 44.5 percent of participants, human resources shortfall was ranked 2nd (37.5 percent), work overload of healthcare workers was ranked

3rd (32 percent), as the factors concerning the key challenges in the implementation of the NHP-2017.

Following recommendations emerge based on the study:

State Health Policy

Given the diversity and complexity of issues at every state, each state must frame its specific policy.

Awareness

Dissemination of information about health policy should happen through an institutionalized mechanism, targeting every stakeholder. Technology platforms, including online media channels, should be effectively utilized.

Communication and Technology

This study clearly indicates the lack of awareness about the national health policies among the masses, and so, there is a need for continuous interaction between the planners, policymakers and the public, and of regular field level studies, for timely and relevant inputs. Technology platforms must be extensively leveraged for timely communication.

Inclusive Approach

Policy inputs must be sought with thematic areas clearly mentioned, for the relevant stakeholders to share inputs. Policymaking must follow a bottom-up approach with inputs from grassroots level workers, beneficiaries, and other appropriate stakeholders. There should be involvement of individual Subject Matter Experts (SMEs), various arms of the government, CSOs, media personnel, academia, and the private sector. This will de-silo the policymaking approach and make it robust.

Quality of Data

Data has been highlighted as another major issue in Indian healthcare. Authentic and updated data is needed for making robust health policies. Epidemiology needs to be strengthened and technology could be extensively used in addressing the issue in totality. With tools of technology available, live data and dashboards should be of immense help in Implementation, Monitoring, and Evaluation. This needs a structured and institutionalized approach with adequate and appropriate human and financial resources.

Evidence-Based Policymaking – Research

Continuous research / field-level surveys are important to get feedback, which is critical for policy formulation, implementation, monitoring, and evaluation. This requires a planned approach as a part of the policymaking process and a partnership between academia, industry, and the government. Evidence should back the policy inputs and formulation.

Capacity Building

Effective policymaking requires capacity building and continuous upskilling of healthcare workers, researchers, and academia. Capacity building is an important prerequisite for effective monitoring and evaluation. Capacity building is also required for the policy formulation process, to ensure that the various components of policymaking are handled by competent professionals.

Impact Assessment – M&E

There is a need for a regular socio-economic audit of the various aspects of health policy in implementation, and suitable amends, as needed, must be made in policy post the field level impact assessment. It is critical to share the key health metrics (with regards to the achievements) with the stakeholders at every level, so that there is a sense of belongingness and ownership in them. Also, it is important to disseminate the findings among the broader network of communities so that ground-level inputs drive the formulation of future health policies through proper engagement and participation at every level.

M&E processes should be automated, and the socioeconomic impact of policies should form the basis of any mid-term policy change.

Formalizing the Policymaking Process

It is time for the government to formalize a policymaking process covering the following:

a) Agenda building and policymaking
b) Planning
c) Implementation
d) Monitoring and Evaluation.

Also, policies and programmes should have a sunset clause. The periodicity (Timelines) of the monitoring and evaluation and policy formulation must be specified, given that the previous health policies have been at irregular intervals. In the age of technology proliferation, health policies should be 'live documents', revised - based on the impact assessment, through monitoring and evaluation, and backed by the real-world evidence.

CPSIA information can be obtained
at www.ICGtesting.com
Printed in the USA
BVHW051432060623
665489BV00014B/741